Research to Action

Research to Action

Structural Racism as a Barrier to Health Equity

Edited by

CLAIRE GIBBONS
ALONZO L. PLOUGH

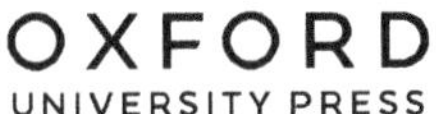

OXFORD
UNIVERSITY PRESS

OXFORD
UNIVERSITY PRESS

Oxford University Press is a department of the University of Oxford.
It furthers the University's objective of excellence in research, scholarship,
and education by publishing worldwide. Oxford is a registered trade mark of
Oxford University Press in the UK and in certain other countries.

Published in the United States of America by Oxford University Press
198 Madison Avenue, New York, NY 10016, United States of America.

Library of Congress Cataloging-in-Publication Data
Names: Gibbons, Claire editor | Plough, Alonzo L. editor |
Robert Wood Johnson Foundation issuing body
Title: Research to action : structural racism as a barrier to health equity /
edited by Claire Gibbons, Alonzo L. Plough.
Description: New York, NY : Oxford University Press, [2026] |
Includes bibliographical references and index.
Identifiers: LCCN 2025044784 (print) | LCCN 2025044785 (ebook) |
ISBN 9780197819845 paperback | ISBN 9780197819852 epub | ISBN 9780197819876
Subjects: LCSH: Racism in medicine—United States | Discrimination in
medical care—United States | Health services accessibility—United States |
Minorities—Medical care—United States | Racism—Health
aspects—United States | United States—Race relations
Classification: LCC RA418.3.U6 R47 2026 (print) | LCC RA418.3.U6 (ebook)
LC record available at https://lccn.loc.gov/2025044784
LC ebook record available at https://lccn.loc.gov/2025044785

DOI: 10.1093/9780197819876.001.0001

The manufacturer's authorized representative in the EU for product safety is
Oxford University Press España S.A. of Parque Empresarial San Fernando de Henares,
Avenida de Castilla, 2 – 28830 Madrid (www.oup.es/en or product.safety@oup.com).
OUP España S.A. also acts as importer into Spain of products made by the manufacturer.

Contents

SECTION III. RESEARCH MEETS COMMUNITY REALITIES: ACTION AND ENGAGEMENT TO CONFRONT STRUCTURAL RACISM

Preface

The nine research papers collected in this book were commissioned by the Robert Wood Johnson Foundation (RWJF) at a time when there was significant and reliable federal support for population health science and interdisciplinary inquiry. At that time, structural determinants research was available, and equity was a goal of federal-level health policies. These papers formed the evidentiary backbone of RWJF's decision to place structural racism at the center of our health equity strategy.

Disturbingly, last year marked a sharp and unprecedented erosion of political, financial, and institutional support for research and policies advancing health equity. What had been a maturing field of inquiry became a target of sustained ideological attack. With the start of the second Trump administration in January 2025, these attacks intensified into an aggressive and coordinated effort to dismantle research on structural racism, health inequity, and the social determinants of health.

A New and Hostile Terrain

We have seen Diversity, Equity, and Inclusion (DEI), reframed not as a set of practices to improve fairness or access, but as an ideological enemy that should be attacked. The administration deployed DEI as a battering ram—a catch-all label used to justify the elimination of scientific programs, research centers, and grant mechanisms that examined racism's impact on health. This was not rhetorical excess; it was a deliberate strategy to delegitimize the empirical study of discrimination, segregation, and structural determinants by depicting them as partisan rather than evidence-based.

Research on racialized health disparities—peer-reviewed, NIH-funded, community-partnered, and long accepted within the public health field—was suddenly categorized as "DEI-driven" and therefore suspect. The goal was clear: if structural racism cannot be named, it cannot be measured; and if it cannot be measured, the nation cannot be held accountable for its consequences.

The Human Costs of Retrenchment

The consequences of these post-2025 actions have been profound. Contributors to this volume and many colleagues across the country have faced threats, loss of funding, and—in some cases—the elimination of their positions as agencies and academic institutions responded to federal pressure.

Graduate students and early-career scholars, particularly scholars of color, are navigating a landscape in which entire research trajectories have become politically precarious. Communities whose lived experiences built the case for structural racism research now face the prospect of losing tools essential to documenting inequities and advocating for change. Weaponizing DEI against population health science has become a mechanism for sustaining the very inequities the research seeks to dismantle.

Why This Research Still Matters

Despite retrenchment, the evidence remains unequivocal: structural racism is one of the most powerful predictors of health across the lifespan. The papers in this volume helped establish that reality with methodological rigor, historical grounding, and a commitment to truth-telling.

The suppression of structural racism research is itself a form of structural racism. It is a refusal to acknowledge the mechanisms that produce inequity, and an attempt to maintain unequal systems by obscuring their operation.

RWJF's Enduring Commitment

In this climate, the RWJF's commitment has not wavered. In 2025, we responded to the attacks on public health by deploying about $10 million in rapid response funding to our grantee partners. As federal structures pulled back, RWJF continued to support rigorous, community-engaged research that names structural racism as a public health crisis. The politicization of DEI is not a neutral policy dispute—it is an obstruction to evidence generation and this nation's pursuit of health equity.

The Foundation's stance is simple: the facts did not change because politics did. The health impacts of structural racism remain measurable, consequential, and central to our nation's future. Advancing health science, grounded in equity, remains essential to dismantling the structural inequities the research was designed to address.

Looking Forward

The attacks on this field have not extinguished it. New generations of scholars, community-driven research networks, and public health practitioners are resilient and continue advancing the work—often drawing directly on foundational insights developed in the papers collected here. RWJF's commitment to research funding remains strong and has expanded to include a new community-connected and equity-focused program called *Health Equity Research for Action*, which will generate evidence to help identify transformative solutions to racial and health inequities.

We present the volume as it was originally conceived, reflecting the historical continuity of evidence-based research on race and health. This current extreme, ideological-driven disruption represents a challenge but not an end to this inquiry. We invite readers to engage not just with the findings, but with the broader question of this current moment: What kind of nation do we become when we fear and disregard the truths our own researchers uncover?

RWJF's conviction remains: a society that confronts structural racism with honesty, rigor, and compassion is one capable of achieving health equity.

Note to the reader: Every chapter was produced by a different research team and therefore the formatting of every chapter is different/inconsistent.

List of Contributors

Salma M. Abdalla, MBBS, MPH, DrPH, is Assistant Professor, Washington University in St. Louis, MO, US.

Chitra Balakrishnan, is Research Analyst at Urban Institute, Washington, DC, US.

Rekha Balu, PhD, is Director, Federal Equity Initiatives at Urban Institute, Washington, DC, US.

Trent Baskerville, MPP, is Research & Technical Assistance Specialist, WestEd Justice & Prevention Research Center, San Francisco, CA, US.

Keisha L. Bentley-Edwards, PhD, is Associate Professor of Medicine, Duke University, Durham, NC, US.

Enobong Hannah "Anna" Branch, PhD, is Senior Vice President for Equity and Professor of Sociology, Rutgers University, New Brunswick, NJ, US.

Lauren Brinkley-Rubinstein, PhD, is Associate Professor, Duke University, Durham, NC, US.

Stephanie Russo Carroll, DrPH, MPH, AB, is Associate Professor, Native Nations Institute, Udall Center for Studies in Public Policy University of Arizona, Tucson, Homelands of the O'odham and contemporary lands of the Yaqui Peoples, AZ, US and Associate Professor, Community, Environment & Policy, Mel and Enid Zuckerman College of Public Health, University of Arizona, Tucson, Homelands of the O'odham and contemporary lands of the Yaqui Peoples, AZ, US.

Tongtan Chantarat, PhD, MPH, is Research Scientist, University of Minnesota School of Public Health, Minneapolis, Minn, US.

Carly Chiwiwi, MD, MPH, is Resident Physician, Department of Family and Community Medicine, Contra Costa Health, Martinez, CA, US.

Liz Contreras is a student, Graduate School of Education, Harvard University, Cambridge, MA, US.

Claire Cusella, MPA, is Senior Policy Program Manager at Urban Institute, Washington, DC, US.

William Darity Jr., PhD, is Visiting Professor of Economics, Howard University, Washington, DC, US.

Nicholas Datto is Research Assistant, The Samuel DuBois Cook Center on Social Equity at Duke University, Durham, NC, US.

Daniel E. Dawes, JD, DHL, Senior Vice President of Global Health and Founding Dean, School of Global Health at Meharry Medical College, Nashville, TN, US.

Jill M. Doerfler, PhD, is Professor and Department Head of American Indian Studies, University of Minnesota Duluth, MN, US.

Shekinah Fashaw-Walters, PhD, Assistant Professor, University of Minnesota School of Public Health, Minneapolis, Minn, US.

Jillian Fish, PhD, MS, is an independent scholar.

CeRon Ford, MPH, Graduate Research Assistant, University of Minnesota School of Public Health, Minneapolis, Minn, US.

Salama S. Freed, MA, PhD, is Assistant Professor of Health Policy and Management, Milken Institute School of Public Health, The George Washington University, Washington, DC, US.

Trevor Fronius, PhD, is Director, WestEd Justice & Prevention Research Center, Newbury, MA, US.

Karishma Furtado, MPH, is Equity Scholar at Urban Institute, Washington, DC, US.

Sandro Galea, MD, DrPH, Dean and Robert A. Knox Professor, Boston University School of Public Health, Boston, MA, US.

Raffi R. Gracia, PhD, MA, Associate Professor of Finance & Accounting, Troy, New York, NY, US and Affiliate Faculty at The Samuel DuBois Cook Center on Social Equity at Duke University, Durham, NC, US.

Joseph P. Gone, PhD, MA, is Professor, Department of Global Health and Social Medicine, Harvard Medical School, Boston, MA, US and Professor, Department of Anthropology, Harvard University, Cambridge, MA, US.

Miigis B. Gonzalez, PhD, MPH, is Assistant Scientist, Johns Hopkins University, Duluth, MN, US.

Tiffany Green, PhD, is Associate Professor, University of Wisconsin-Madison, Madison, Wisconsin, US.

Rachel Hardeman, PhD, MPH, is Professor, University of Minnesota School of Public Health, Minneapolis, Minn, US.

Anna K. Hing, PhD, MPH, is Research Scientist, University of Minnesota School of Public Health, Minneapolis, Minn, US.

Michelle Kahn-John, PhD, is Assistant Professor, Johns Hopkins, Baltimore, MD, US.

Candance King, PhD, is Research Director and Project Manager, Black Bodies Black Health Research Project, Rutgers University, New Brunswick, NJ, US.

Tonya (Connor) Kjerland, MS, is a PhD candidate, University of North Dakota, Grand Forks, MN, US.

Cosette Lias, MPP, is Research Assistant, WestEd Justice & Prevention Research Center, San Francisco, CA, US.

Pamela MacDougall is Research Assistant, WestEd Justice & Prevention Research Center, Woburn, MA, US.

Morgan Maner, MSc, is Project Coordinator, The University of North Carolina at Chapel Hill School of Medicine, Chapel Hill, NC, US.

Tara L. Maudrie, PhD, MSPH, is Assistant Professor, School of Social Work, University of Michigan, Ann Arbor, MI, US.

Jennifer Messenger is Senior Executive Vice President, Public Health, Metropolitan Group, Portland, OR, US.

Raquel Motachwa, MPH, Research Assistant, University of Minnesota School of Public Health, Minneapolis, Minn, US.

Danielle Munguia, MS, is Research Assistant, WestEd Justice & Prevention Research Center, Los Angeles, CA, US.

Ericka C. Muñoz, MS, is Research Assistant, WestEd Justice & Prevention Research Center, Irvine, CA, US.

Victoria M. O'Keefe, PhD, MS, is Associate Professor, Department of International Health, Center for Indigenous Health, Johns Hopkins Bloomberg School of Public Health, Johns Hopkins University, Baltimore, MD, US.

Tori O'Neal, MA, is Principal Consultant at O'Neal Consulting, Silver Spring, MD, US.

Myra Parker, JD, MPH, PhD, is Associate Professor, University of Washington, Seattle, WA, US.

Surili Sutaria Patel, MS, is Vice President, Public Health, Metropolitan Group, Portland, OR, US.

Anthony Petrosino, PhD, is Senior Fellow, George Mason University Center for Evidence-based Crime Policy, Alexandria, VA, US.

Leigha Puckett, MS, is Research Associate, WestEd Justice & Prevention Research Center, Washington, DC, US.

Thomas D. Sequist, MD, MPH, is Professor, Medicine and Health Care Policy, Harvard Medical School, Boston, MA, US and Chief Patient Experience and Equity Officer, Mass General Brigham, Boston, MA, US.

Arjumand Siddiqi, ScD, is Professor and Canada Research Chair in Population Health Equity, University of Toronto, Toronto, Ontario, Canada.

Michelle Stephens, PhD, LP, is Psychoanalytic Teaching Faculty, William Alanson White Institute of Psychiatry, Psychoanalysis and Psychology, Manhattan, NY, US; Professor of English and Latino and Caribbean Studies, Rutgers University, New Brunswick, NJ, US; and Founding and Executive Director, Institute for the Study of Global Racial Justice (ISGRJ), Rutgers University, New Brunswick, NJ, US.

Angelia Turner, MS, is Senior Equity Lead in Justice, WestEd Justice & Prevention Research Center, San Francisco, CA, US and Director, Richland County Criminal Justice Coordinating Council, Columbia, South Carolina, US.

Melissa L. Walls, PhD, is Professor of American Health; Co-Director, Johns Hopkins University, Center for Indigenous Health, Baltimore, MD, US.

Rachel E. Wilbur, PhD, MPH, is Research Assistant Professor, Department of Medical Education and Clinical Sciences, IREACH Program, Elson S. Floyd College of Medicine, Washington State University, Spokane, WA, US.

Introduction

We now have abundant evidence that structural racism is a ubiquitous social force that shapes health in the United States. However, despite this growing recognition, structural racism and its influence on health outcomes have received insufficient research attention. As recently as 2018, a comprehensive literature review revealed that only 20 articles had been published on the topic over the previous three decades.[1]

The increased recognition that racism, rather than simply race, is the driving force behind many health disparities has dramatically increased the number of studies and publications focused on a host of interrelated issues. As researchers, philanthropies, journals, and community organizations recognize the urgency of understanding structural racism[2] and health in all its complexity, there are many new efforts to build that knowledge base. While research that identifies structural racism as an influence on health outcomes *and* links to useful action is still scant, the body of evidence crucial to informing action continues to grow.

This volume makes an important contribution by presenting different approaches to defining structural racism and closely examining the pathways through which structural racism creates health inequities—and then going further with concrete ideas for addressing and redressing this problem. It unpacks the assumptions that influence research methodology and mindsets and looks hard at the damage wrought by the criminal justice system, the structure of political systems, the distortions imposed by wealth disparities, the enduring impact of colonialism, the intertwined relationship between climate and health, and more. This type of research is deliberately

---

[1] Groos et al. Measuring inequity: A systematic review of methods used to quantify structural racism. *Journal of Health Disparities Research and Practice.* 2019;11(2):18. https://digitalscholarship.unlv.edu/jhdrp/vol11/iss2/13/.

[2] Structural racism is race-based unfair treatment built into policies, laws, and practices. It is also called "systemic" racism because it is fostered through mutually reinforcing systems, policies, and practices in housing, education, employment, earnings, benefits, credit, media, health care, and criminal justice. These patterns and practices reinforce discriminatory beliefs, values, and the distribution of resources, which all effect health.

Claire Gibbons and Alonzo L. Plough, *Introduction.* In: *Research to Action.* Edited by: Claire Gibbons and Alonzo L. Plough, Oxford University Press. © Robert Wood Johnson Foundation (2026).
DOI: 10.1093/9780197819876.003.0001

cross-disciplinary, recognizing the imperative of considering common challenges through the lenses of better integrated and connected scholarship and practice to advance informed solutions. It is also partnered with and inclusive of the ideas and experiences of persons who experience marginalized conditions in their communities.

The Robert Wood Johnson Foundation (RWJF) is a leader *and* a learner in this work. We have long been engaged in the push for greater health equity, building on the principle that much of what drives health happens outside clinical settings and that community power promotes change.[3] Some of our most direct and vigorous commitments can be traced back to the Commission to Build a Healthier America, which we formed in 2013 to consider how the places we live, work, learn, and play influence our health. The Commission's 10 recommendations, published in *Time to Act: Investing in the Health of Our Children and Communities*,[4] set the stage for both the social determinants focus and the Culture of Health agenda that RWJF has pursued for more than a decade.

Recognizing the central role of social determinants in health and the challenge of health inequities in marginalized communities, we focus our investments in priority areas that include transformative change in public health and health care systems, healthy community conditions, thriving children and families, and supporting community capacity and power to lead changes designed to improve health equity. In our grantmaking and partnership-building activities, we are committed to expanding and sharing the data, knowledge, and tools that will help America transform into a society where health is no longer a privilege, but a right.

In the years since RWJF began digging into the root causes of unfair health outcomes, the realities of structural racism have become ever more apparent to us. Through discussion, partnerships, and grantmaking, we have sought to clarify our own role in eliminating them and to enrich our understanding of the experiences and innovative ideas generated from the lived experience of minoritized groups. Our efforts have been informed by the scholarship of experts and by the lived experience of individuals and communities with whom RWJF had not previously engaged.

---

[3] RWJF. *Building community power to advance health equity.* https://www.rwjf.org/en/our-vision/focus-areas.html

[4] RWJF. *Commission to build a healthier America.* http://www.commissiononhealth.org/.

Widening our circle has allowed us to forge new connections and cemented our own determination to be a catalyst for creating conditions in which all can thrive. We are not, of course, alone in doing so. The murder of George Floyd, only the most highly publicized and visually documented in the continuous history of unjust police killings of Black people, sparked national protests and set off a long overdue national conversation about race. The disparities exacerbated by the COVID-19 pandemic were another clear example of the link between structural racism and poor health outcomes.

All of this accelerated our focus on structural racism at RWJF. Our research and evidence-based evaluations, including analyzing a deep body of externally developed and funded evidence, allows us to elucidate the mutually reinforcing policies, laws, and practices that buttress discriminatory beliefs, values, and uneven resource distribution. As we move deeper into this work, we have become less focused on defining the problem or further documenting disparities, and more intent on listening closely to the affected communities and embracing bold action toward systematic changes that eliminate the effects of structural racism on health outcomes.

RWJF-funded initiatives such as Finding Answers: Disparities Research for Change,[5] Interdisciplinary Research Leaders,[6] and the National Commission to Transform Public Health Data Systems[7] are among the many vehicles we are using to drive change. By layering rigorous research alongside the passion and resolve bubbling up in so many communities across the country, these multi-pronged collaborations take direct aim at the systems and structures that allow racism to endure. We are also encouraging interventions to close the racial wealth gap for families and communities through our Policies for Action (P4A) program,[8] funding studies of guaranteed income (for example, evaluating the Stockton Economic Empowerment Demonstration[9] and supporting the Center for Guaranteed Income Research[10]), and considering how best to employ asset-building strategies from baby bonds and tax incentives to reparations.

---

[5] RWJF. *Finding answers: Disparities research for change.* http://forces4quality.org/.

[6] RWJF. *Interdisciplinary research leaders.* https://irleaders.org/.

[7] RWJF. *National commission to transform public health data systems.* https://www.rwjf.org/en/insights/our-research/2021/09/transforming-public-health-data-systems.html.

[8] RWJF. 2022. *P4A call for proposals.* https://anr.rwjf.org/viewCfp.do?cfpId=1644&cfpOverviewId=

[9] Stockton Economic Empowerment Demonstration. https://www.evidenceforaction.org/grant/volatility-agency-and-health-city-led-guaranteed-income-experiment.

[10] Center for Guaranteed Income Research, University of Pennsylvania. https://www.penncgir.org/

This work is taking place at a fractured moment in American society, a time of tremendous pushback against equity-building strategies. Some of our grantees have told us that having necessary conversations about the impact of racism on health outcomes has led to vicious attempts to undermine their work.

We need to take an objective look at the clear evidence of health disparities experienced in marginalized communities and to consider their source. It is simply not possible to understand American history without exploring the fact of racism that is woven through it.

Communicating that message is essential to our commitments at RWJF. In 2022, we published *Necessary Conversations: Understanding Racism as a Barrier to Achieving Health Equity*,[11] recommended by STAT as "a must-read," and "a deeply powerful and impressively original look at the roots of racial health inequities in America."[12] RWJF leaders are speaking out about the many issues that intersect with structural racism, publishing opinion pieces and commenting on proposed regulations related to fair housing,[13] safe drinking water,[14] nondiscrimination in health programs,[15] inequities in medical practice,[16] the right to child care,[17] and much more.

At the same time, we recognize that there is much more for us to learn. So recent is societal attention to structural racism that the term itself has yet to be consistently defined. The complexity of conducting research has been further compounded by decades in which the agenda has been set largely by a limited group of academic scholars, to the exclusion of community voices. The result is a failure to interrogate some of the core methodological

[11] Plough AL, ed. *Necessary conversations: Understanding racism as a barrier to achieving health equity.* Oxford University Press.

[12] Mupo S. The 27 best books and podcasts on health and science to check out this summer. *STAT.* July 5, 2023. https://www.statnews.com/2023/07/05/summer-book-podcast-list-beach-reads-2023/.

[13] Besser R. Affirmatively furthering fair housing proposed rule. April 24, 2023. https://www.rwjf.org/en/insights/advocacy-and-policy/regulatory-comments/2023/04/comments-from-richard-besser-on-affirmatively-furthering-fair-housing-proposed-rule.html.

[14] Morita, J. Finally, a chance to get the lead out nationwide. *Governing.* May 30, 2023. https://www.governing.com/health/finally-a-chance-to-get-the-lead-out-nationwide.

[15] Besser, R. Nondiscrimination in health programs and activities proposed rule. October 3, 2022. https://www.rwjf.org/en/insights/advocacy-and-policy/regulatory-comments/2022/10/comments-from-richard-besser-on-nondiscrimination-in-health-programs-and-activities-proposed-rule.html.

[16] Lavizzo-Mourey RJ, Besser, RE, Willilams, DR. Understanding and mitigating health inequities: Past, current, and future directions. *New England Journal of Medicine.* 2021;384: 1681–1684. doi:10.1056/NEJMp2008628.

[17] Morita J. America's broken child care system deserves a permanent fix. *The Hill.* September 5, 2023. https://thehill.com/opinion/education/4186441-americas-broken-child-care-system-deserves-a-permanent-fix/.

assumptions that exclude essential information drawn from actual community contexts. One RWJF initiative to address that limitation is Transforming Academia for Equity, which funds university-based public health schools and programs to create a culture in which underrepresented researchers can thrive.[18]

In 2022, RWJF commissioned a series of papers to inform its future grant-making strategy. Deliberately reaching beyond our established networks, we sought out contributors from diverse fields, many of whom brought not only innovative thinking to their scholarship but also insights gained from personal experiences with structural racism. Such was the power of the resulting work that we felt it demanded a broader audience. This book, organized in three sections, is the result.

- **Section I** presents evidence of how structural racism influences health. A vigorous literature review, a look at how politics and policy determine the distribution of resources and power, and a blunt discussion of wealth disparities by race set the stage for moving forward.
- **Section II** dives into upstream knowledge-building strategies for gathering actionable data and explores the systemic changes that can produce equitable health outcomes. The limits of the existing body of knowledge demand innovative new strategies and inclusive information-gathering approaches that are explored here.
- **Section III** primarily focuses on the use of research to generate action. The contributors consider how best to understand and chip away at bias within the criminal justice arena, position indigenous health challenges within the context of colonial subjugation, use the lens of humanistic and social science to counter stigmatizing cultural images of Black bodies, and highlight community power as a tool for confronting climate change.

While there is much here to inform the work of researchers, policymakers, funders, and community activists, it is important to acknowledge that these chapters are not comprehensive. In particular, issues affecting the Latino and Asian populations are not specifically addressed, nor are the challenges associated with immigration, although RWJF does make significant grants in these areas.

---

[18] RWJF. *Call for proposals, Transforming academia for equity.* https://anr.rwjf.org/viewCfp.do?cfpId=1606%cfpOverviewId.

In a rapidly evolving field, we make no pretense of having all the answers. The road ahead is long, the next steps are not always obvious, and the measures, methods, and definitions needed to translate data seamlessly into interventions remain incomplete. But we know enough to make progress. At this pivotal moment, we must be bold. We cannot substitute nomenclature and rhetoric for analysis. It is equally imperative to move past labels and slogans, accept ambiguity and acknowledge nuance, test and revise new approaches, and base action on evidence broadly conceived. The ideas and information in this volume inspire us at RWJF to continue thinking ever more carefully about our role and responsibility to serve equity.

Building Community Power to Advance Health Equity

How do local community power-building organizations advance health and racial equity?

For more than 20 years, the Robert Wood Johnson Foundation (RWJF) has supported community power organizations and advocacy networks that engage in grassroots organizing, particularly with people who are low-income, of color, and/or youths. The Foundation has supported communities in their power-building efforts to mitigate tobacco use and childhood obesity and, most recently, to improve community conditions and confront structural racism.

Elevating Community Power and Community Voice

We all have dreams for ourselves and our families. But we don't all have the same opportunities to make those dreams come true. Structural barriers and systemic racism are persistent obstacles to achieving health equity. Black, Indigenous, and People of Color are leading vital movements that are galvanizing their communities and seeding transformative change. Building and bridging power within communities is essential to the health and well-being of people who have endured decades of racial injustice, economic exclusion, social marginalization, and health inequities.

Low-income people and communities of color have been excluded from decision-making on the policies and practices that impact their health and prosperity, through generations of systemic exclusion and disinvestment. Our learning has shown that the people most directly affected by systemic barriers and inequities are best positioned to identify the solutions and actions needed to drive change.

That's why community power is important to how RWJF contributes to transformative change, in a variety of areas—from housing, to healthcare, to birthing, to family caregiving. The evaluation of this work, which will center on the principles of equitable evaluation, should begin to shed light on the impact we can have in community power-building and support our learning efforts to hone our strategies.

To learn more about RWJF's strategies in this area, visit www.rwjf.org.

GETTING TO THE ROOT: BUILDING ACTIONABLE EVIDENCE ABOUT STRUCTURAL RACISM'S IMPACT ON HEALTH

Section I lays the groundwork for exploring opportunities to dismantle one of society's greatest ills. Until recently, studies of the decisive role that underlying structural racism plays in explaining differing health indicators across populations and zip codes were sparse. The rise of Black Lives Matter and other social change movements, coupled with impossible-to-ignore markers of inequity during the COVID-19 pandemic, changed that dynamic. The three chapters in this part document racial inequities, identify root causes, and widen the lens through which to consider the distribution of harm. Special consideration is given to the role that political structures and wealth play in influencing health outcomes.

Chapter 1, Mapping the Literature on the Effects of Structural Racism on Health Outcomes in the United States: A Path Forward examines a decade of published research (2011–2021) at the intersection of structural racism and the health inequities that sicken and kill. The review covers the broad topics of education, employment and financial strain, healthcare access and quality, the built environment, and the judicial system. While acknowledging that current knowledge is limited, that grounding informs a package of recommendations to undercut structural racism and improve health. These are framed around four strategies: advocating for structural changes, developing and testing interventions that can be scaled up, catalyzing a national conversation, and investing in research.

Chapter 2, Political Determinants of Racial Inequities in Health and the Race Against Policy-Related Inequities and Determinants (RAPID) travels upstream to explore the political action, inaction, and decision-making that lead to inequity. This analytical approach recognizes that the ways in which relationships are structured, resources are distributed, and power is administered reflect systemic processes that need to be interrogated to support change. Within this conceptual framework, a strategy for integrating health equity into the plans, programs, and organizational culture at every level of government and in community-serving organizations can flourish. To sharpen opportunities for positive impact, the political determinants of health are considered across five intersecting domains: voting, government, policy, advocacy, and commercial interests.

Chapter 3, Health, Wealth, and Structural Racism: Interconnected Drivers of Racial Health Disparities documents the differences in wealth accumulation between Black and White people and how that shapes health outcomes across generations. Asset gaps, reflected particularly in home ownership and savings accounts, are the product of countless racist policies, including land seizures, redlining, the administration of GI Bill benefits, the destruction of Black business districts, and the failure to make restitution for slavery. A fuller understanding of how the racial wealth gap influences health requires incorporating race as a social construct into research design and disaggregating data to pinpoint differing outcomes. Of the many policies explored in this chapter to boost Black wealth and confront racism within the healthcare system, reparations are recognized as the boldest and most direct bridging strategy.

1

Mapping the Literature on the Effects of Structural Racism on Health Outcomes in the United States: A Path Forward

Salma M. Abdalla and Sandro Galea

Structural Racism and Racial/Ethnic Health Disparities in the United States

Structural racism has created barriers to opportunity for a significant proportion of the United States population since the nation's founding. The disenfranchisement has taken many forms throughout American history and ranges from discrimination in formal systems, such as slavery and Jim Crow laws, to practices, such as redlining and segregation, all of which contributed to the marginalization of whole groups, particularly Black Americans and Native Americans. The deep and persistent racial and ethnic health gaps observed today emerge directly from this disenfranchisement and attendant foreshortening of economic and social opportunities for racial and ethnic minority groups in the country.

There is no single agreed-upon definition of structural racism or other related terms such as systemic or institutional racism. As Table 1.1 shows, a range of definitions by different scholars offers multiple perspectives that often emphasize how structural racism embeds discrimination against persons based on their membership of a particular racial or ethnic group in all aspects of regulatory and normative frameworks. Definitions also emphasize that structural racism is the product of centuries of laws, practices, economic systems, and societal norms that ultimately shape the country.[1] We will use this overarching understanding of structural racism throughout this chapter.

Salma M. Abdalla and Sandro Galea, *Mapping the Literature on the Effects of Structural Racism on Health Outcomes in the United States: A Path Forward*. In: *Research to Action*. Edited by: Claire Gibbons and Alonzo L. Plough, Oxford University Press. © Robert Wood Johnson Foundation (2026).
DOI: 10.1093/9780197819876.003.0002

Table 1.1 A selection of definitions of structural racism and other relevant terms

Term	Definition
Structural racism	"Structural racism involves interconnected institutions, whose linkages are historically rooted and culturally reinforced. It refers to the totality of ways in which societies foster racial discrimination, through mutually reinforcing inequitable systems (in housing, education, employment, earnings, benefits, credit, media, health care, criminal justice, and so on) that in turn reinforce discriminatory beliefs, values, and distribution of resources, which together affect the risk of adverse health outcomes."[38]
	"Structural racism is defined as the macrolevel systems, social forces, institutions, ideologies, and processes that interact with one another to generate and reinforce inequities among racial and ethnic groups . . . [s]tructural mechanisms do not require the actions or intent of individuals."[39]
	"A system in which public policies, institutional practices, cultural representations, and other norms work in various, often reinforcing ways to perpetuate racial group inequity."[40]
Institutional racism	"Racially adverse 'discriminatory policies and practices carried out . . . [within and between individual] state or non-state institutions' on the basis of racialised group membership."[38,41]
Environmental racism	"a form of systemic racism whereby communities of color are disproportionately burdened with health hazards through policies and practices"[42]
Residential segregation	"The geographic separation of racial groups' homes [neighborhoods, and communities]."[39]
Redlining	"the practice of mortgage lending discrimination based on racial neighborhood composition and purposeful financial disinvestment in non-white neighborhoods ('red zones')"[43]
Intergenerational drag	The "intergenerational drag hypothesis posits that 'Ethnic or racial groups pass social assets and liabilities on to their descendants' . . . the cumulative effects of macrolevel systems interacting with one another in ways that generate and sustain racial inequalities."[39]
Jim Crow	"The segregation and disenfranchisement laws known as 'Jim Crow' represented a formal, codified system of racial apartheid that dominated the American South for three quarters of a century beginning in the 1890s."[44]
Black codes	"[I]n U.S. history, any of numerous laws enacted in the states of the former Confederacy after the American Civil War and intended to assure the continuance of white supremacy."[45]

Structural Racism and the Forces that Shape Health

The impact of structural racism is felt in all aspects of American life. For example, in 2018–2019 American Indian/Alaska Native persons had the lowest percentage (74%) of public high school students graduating four years from starting 9th grade, followed by Black (80%), Hispanic (82%), White (89%) and Asian (93%) persons.[2] College enrollment rates in 2019 reflected similar patterns. The percentage of Asian (89.9%) and White (66.9%) students enrolling in postsecondary education were higher than Hispanic (63.4%) and Black (50.7%) students. When it comes to earnings, in 2019, the median annual salary of White workers ($76,057) was above that of Hispanic ($56,113) and Black ($46,073) workers.[3]

Racial and ethnic disparities exist in access to, and quality of, the built environment as well. The percentage of homeownership among Black Americans at the start of 2021 (45.1%) has not improved upon what it was in 1966 (46%) and remains far below the homeownership percentage of White Americans in 2021 (73.8%).[4,5] These rates can be understood in the context of the policies and practices that have long affected homeownership. In 2015, denial rates of conventional loans for one-to-four family homes were highest for Black applicants (27.4%), followed by Hispanic (19.2%), White (10.9%), and Asian (10.8%) applicants.[6] Even when a mortgage is approved, Black and Hispanic buyers often pay more than their White and Asian counterparts. Black and Hispanic payers also consistently make up the majority of payers for higher mortgage rates than their White counterparts and the percentage of Black payers at the mortgage rate of 8% or higher were nearly double all other groups.[6]

The judicial system is one of the country's structures with the highest disparities by racial and ethnic group. One in three Black men and one in seven Hispanic men will face imprisonment at some point in their lives, compared to one in 17 White men.[7,8] Black men are three times as likely and Hispanic men are 2.5 times as likely to be incarcerated as White men.[7] This is despite different racial and ethnic groups having comparable crime rates for certain offenses. For example, drug use rates do not differ significantly by racial and ethnic group. However, in 2015, more than one in four persons arrested for violation of drug laws was Black.[9]

Similar disparities exist in the healthcare system. As of 2020, Hispanic (26.5%) adults between 18 and 64 had the greatest uninsured rates, followed by Black (13.2%), White (9.7%), and Asian (9.3%) adults in the US.[10]

In terms of quality of care, in 2019, the National Healthcare Quality and Disparities Report showed that Black and American Indian/Alaska Native patients received worse care than White patients for about 40 percent of quality measures, and Hispanic patients received worse care than White patients for about a third of quality measures.[11]

Racial and Ethnic Health Disparities in the United States

Given the racial and ethnic inequities in the forces that shape health—such as education, the built environment, the judicial system, and access to and quality of healthcare—it follows that racial and ethnic disparities in health would be ubiquitous in the United States.

Overall, minority groups consistently have lower life expectancy than their White counterparts. They also face a higher risk of non-communicable diseases and their antecedents, including obesity, diabetes, heart disease, and stroke. By way of example, in 2020, the life expectancy dropped for all racial and ethnic groups coincident with the COVID-19 pandemic. However, the life expectancy of Black Americans dropped far more than it did for White Americans. The gap between life expectancy for Black and White persons widened from 4.1 years in 2019 to 5.8 years in 2020.[12]

Recognizing the ubiquity of structural racism and the attendant ubiquity of racial and ethnic inequities in health raises the question: how do we map the relation between structural racism and health indicators? Insofar as structural racism is everywhere, and shapes all the forces around us, it is difficult to articulate simple linear relations between structural racism and health. Therefore, despite—or perhaps because of—its ubiquity, our understanding of how structural racism influences the conditions we live in and shapes our health, remains in its infancy. Even more so, the academic literature dedicated to locating the key inflection points for interventions intended to mitigate the impact of structural racism on health, though extensive, is underdeveloped. Structural racism has posed a challenge for academia to operationally define and empirically measure, because studies often focus on more accessible perceived racism at the individual and interpersonal levels.[13–17]

Recently, however, there have been increasing efforts—particularly by researchers from groups historically underrepresented in academia—to understand and address the impact of structural racism on health in the

United States. We provide multiple examples of such reviews in Table 1.2. A careful read of these reviews suggests that there is increasing consensus that a holistic understanding of racial and ethnic health inequities can best be understood by focusing on the specific pathways that may link structural racism and health.

Chapter Objectives and Methods

In this chapter, we build on these existing efforts and aim to map relevant peer-reviewed literature published between 2011 and 2021 that describe the intersection between structural racism in five areas—education, employment and financial strain, healthcare access and quality, the built environment, and the judicial system—and health inequities in 10 major causes of morbidity and mortality in the United States. The health outcomes assessed include accidents and unintentional injury, asthma, cancers, cardiovascular diseases, COVID-19, diabetes, HIV/AIDS, life expectancy, mental health, maternal mortality, and obesity.

The results presented in this chapter should be interpreted with a number of considerations in mind. First, given its ubiquity, structural racism, to some degree or another, accounts for "everything." This includes inequities in wealth and income, which then have an impact on almost all other forces that shape health. We acknowledge that this may present challenges to efforts to understand the full role of structural racism in shaping health. Second, the racial and ethnic groupings used in the literature are neither permanent nor fully inclusive, especially when used to unpack the role structural racism has in shaping health outcomes. Third, and importantly, scientific inquiry does not exist in vacuum, and the questions being asked and answered in the literature emerge from a system that is itself shaped by structural racism.

With these considerations in mind, we aimed to offer a systematic effort at characterizing the links between structural racism and health inequities, building on the established understanding of the principal pathways that embed structural racism into the American experience. The results presented in this chapter are based on 75 empirical studies that explicitly used a structural racism framing to assess racial and ethnic health inequities. The chapter also provides empirical evidence of how inequities in education (14 studies), employment and financial strain (11 studies), healthcare access and quality (107 studies), the built environment (141 studies), and the judicial system (11 studies) shape racial/ethnic health inequities.

Table 1.2 Summary of relevant conceptual and literature review efforts

Author/year	Study objectives	Key findings	Themes
Conceptual articles			
Gee GC et al. (2011)[39]	To review different ways of conceptualizing structural racism.	• Social segregation is embedded in housing, schools, workplaces, and healthcare facilities. It functions to concentrate poverty, pollutants, other adverse conditions. • Segregation of social circles leads to racialized patterns of infectious disease spread. • Intergenerational drag (cumulation and passing of racial disparities across time/generation) shows that past events have consequences for following generations.	• Focuses on structural, institutional racism. • Considers structural racism a fundamental cause of health inequities. • Focuses on three dimensions of structural racism: (1) social segregation, (2) immigration policy, (3) intergenerational effects.
Reskin (2012)[46]	To conceptualize the reciprocal interdependence of racial disparities across domains as a "race discrimination system" by using a systems perspective and to discuss possible remedies for systematic racial disparities that stem from a systems perspective.	• Systems perspective: The components of systems are linked through reciprocal causation (i.e., feedback loops) and are inherently dynamic. • A race discrimination system exists if three conditions are met: (1) race-linked disparities exist in every subsystem, (2) at least some of these disparities result directly from discrimination, (3) disparities in each subsystem are reciprocally linked to disparities in other subsystems. • Uber (or meta) discrimination is an emergent form of discrimination that influences the cultural and social contexts in which people act and distorts how others are seen, the attributions made about them, and predictions of their performance. • Discrimination exists within subsystems, reciprocal feedback occurs between subsystems.	• Focuses on structural, institutional racism. • Importance of applying systems perspective when discussing discrimination/racism. • Argument against reductionism: cannot break discrimination/racism down to its constituent parts and analyze in isolation. • Interconnected nature of discrimination systems—reciprocal feedback between subsystems results in accumulation of White privilege and Black disadvantage. • Within each subsystem (1) racial disparities favor Whites, (2) ongoing race discrimination is implicated in the disparities, (3) disparities are causally interdependent across subsystems.

		• Leverage points are points in a subsystem that are essential for system maintenance.	• Two methods to intervene and dismantle race discrimination systems: (1) utilize leverage points in subsystems that are essential for the continued existence of the system and/or (2) the introduction of an exogenous force that acts simultaneously on all of its subsystems.
Bailey ZD et al. (2017)[1]	To examine what constitutes structural racism, generate evidence of how structural racism harms health, and describe interventions that can reduce its impact.	• Structural racism and institutional racism have distinct meanings. • "Color blind" racism in government policies may not be explicitly racist but targets certain groups. • Racism operates in the private sector, particularly in housing and employment. • Racism-health pathways include (1) economic/social deprivation, (2) environmental/occupational inequity, (3) psychosocial trauma, (4) targeted marketing of unhealthy substances, (5) inadequate healthcare, (6) state-sanctioned violence, (7) political exclusion, (8) maladaptive coping behaviors, (9) stereotype threat. • Focuses on structural racism's adverse health impact through two pathways: residential segregation and healthcare quality and access. • Potential solutions include (1) place-based initiatives create structures for reinvesting in sidelined neighborhoods, (2) policy changes in government sentencing/incarceration, (3) education for healthcare professionals on structural competency, cultural humility, and cultural safety.	• Focuses on structural, institutional racism. • Multiple dimensions of structural racism, interconnected and reinforcing inequitable structures. • Structural racism is historically rooted, culturally reinforced. • Multiple direct and indirect pathways between racism and health. • Historically de jure or explicit policies and culture of racism have transitioned into de facto or unspoken racism in government, private institutions, and public culture. De facto and de jure racism both impact the marginalized. • Intersectoral work, targeted interventions are needed to address systemic racism, but the interconnected nature of structural racism necessitates multiple points of intervention.

continued

Table 1.2 *continued*

Author/year	Study objectives	Key findings	Themes
O'Brien R et al. (2020)[47]	To provide population health researchers with a new empirical tool and analytic framework for examining structural racism's influence on generating racial health disparities.	• There is a positive association between ROG and RMG across US counties. • For males, moving from the 25th percentile of the ROG to the 75th percentile is associated with an increase of 85 per 100,000 deaths. • For females, moving from the 25th percentile of the ROG to the 75th percentile is associated with an increase of 50 per 100,000 deaths. • The coefficient on ROG remains statistically significant even after inclusion of covariates and regardless of weighting schema.	• ROG measures the underlying, often obscured effect of place in disparities between SES and health outcomes. • ROG cannot pinpoint the specific disparity that impacts a health outcome in a given place, as these aspects likely vary by locality. • ROG lacks granularity as to specific health outcomes, especially non-fatal ones and only accounts for trends in mortality. • ROG is a retrospective measure of place and is constructed based on the mobility outcomes for cohorts born in the early 1980s. • ROG will be useful in spatial or place-based analyses of racism. • Can serve as an analytic/quantitative measure to supplement place-based analyses.

| Adkins-Jackson PB et al. (2021)[48] | To inspire use of up-to-date and theoretically driven approaches to increase discourse among researchers on measuring racism, as well as improve evidence of its role as the fundamental cause of racial health inequities. | <ul><li>Single dimension measures of structural racism do not capture its multidimensional nature and the extent to which numerous institutions and sectors reinforce health inequities.</li><li>Race is a social construct with no basis in biological or cultural differences between groups; significant differences between races are the result of social exclusion and differences in treatment, rather than inherent biological or cultural differences.</li><li>To determine variables of interest/relation, epidemiologists should engage with interdisciplinary scholars. Sociology, ethnic/culture studies scholars can determine structural factors and individual outcomes, and legal scholars can determine structural factors and health outcomes.</li><li>Few datasets exist with multilevel/multidimensional structural racism measures; epidemiologists need to link existing databases using anchor variables.</li><li>Mixed methods analyses provide empirical statistics and context-based descriptions and allow for a complete picture of SDOH.</li><li>Life-course approach and time sensitive analysis assess exposure during sensitive and critical periods, cumulative exposures, other exposures, and their combinations.</li><li>Researcher reflexivity, a process whereby individuals examine and discuss their beliefs, should be incorporated by researchers and epidemiologists.</li><li>Structural equation models can holistically capture intricacies of policies and practices that are influenced by structural racism.</li></ul> | <ul><li>Focuses on structural, institutional racism.</li><li>Race is not equivalent to structural racism.</li><li>Many measures of structural racism often consider a single dimension in isolation.</li><li>Study of structural racism and health effects requires input from across many fields.</li><li>Structural barriers in academia and publishing prevent or reduce research on structural racism as a cause of health.</li><li>Mixed methods analysis and life course approaches are recommended.</li><li>Structural racism is mutable over time</li><li>Potential issue of collinearity when using multidimensional models with interrelated factors of structural racism; recommend compiling multiple dimensions of structural racism into an index of variables or a latent construct.</li></ul> |

continued

Table 1.2 *continued*

Author/year	Study objectives	Key findings	Themes
Yearby R et al. (2021)[49]	To determine what jurisdictions are working with national racial equity tool organizations, particularly GARE and/or PolicyLink; to determine whether these jurisdictions are enacting or modifying laws to address systemic racism and SDOH; to understand whether and how working with racial equity tool organizations resulted in governmental changes that address systemic racism and SDOH.	• 107 jurisdictions are working with GARE and/or PolicyLink. • Jurisdictions using racial equity tools are located throughout the country and vary widely. • Jurisdictions using racial equity tools were at the forefront of declaring racism as a public health crisis and have enacted or revised minimum wage laws to address SDOH. • Working with GARE and/or PolicyLink resulted in governmental changes in strategic planning, training, workplace practices, and other laws and policies.	• Systemic racism and inequities in SDOH are a result of centuries of inequality and are not random. They will take generations to actively dismantle and address. • Jurisdictions should use a racial equity framework that clearly articulates racial equity, implicit and explicit bias, and individual, institutional, and structural racism.

Literature review

Corral I et al. (2015)[50]	To summarize findings of the residential racial segregation and body weight among African American adults literature in an effort to elucidate the segregation–obesity relationship.	• Positive relationship between segregation and BMI/obesity/overweight; (8 out of 11 studies). • Only 4 of the 11 studies used valid measures of both segregation and overweight/obesity and also controlled for area-poverty.	• Inconsistencies in study results by and large reflect inconsistencies in their measures and their control of neighborhood-SES. • Studies tended to find a positive relationship if they used valid measures of segregation and of over-weight/obesity. • Future studies should use valid measures of segregation and of overweight/obesity to clarify the relationship between them and potentially enhance prevention efforts.
Kershaw KN et al. (2015)[51]	To summarize findings in the segregation and cardiovascular health literature for Blacks and Hispanics, discuss the implications of these findings for racial/ethnic CVD disparities, and identify knowledge gaps.	• Studies of Black residential segregation suggest higher metropolitan-level Black segregation is associated with worse CVD risk. • The majority of neighborhood-level segregation studies also showed higher segregation was related to worse CVD risk, but findings were more mixed. • Relationships among Hispanics were more mixed and appeared to vary widely by factors such as gender, country of origin, racial identity, and acculturation.	• Broader focus on CVD risk factors may identify the pathways linking segregation to disparities in CVD outcomes. • Prospective studies of segregation and CVD risk are needed to understand how persistent exposure to segregation, as well as changes in exposure over the life course, influence CVD risk. • Objective measurement of CVD risk will strengthen the validity of study findings, but increased validity may come at the expense of generalizability of findings. • Integration of social theory is needed to support the measures chosen to assess segregation. • Consider heterogeneity of associations within race/ethnic groups.

continued

Table 1.2 *continued*

Author/year	Study objectives	Key findings	Themes
Paradies Y et al. (2015)[13]	To review the literature on the relationship between reported racism and mental and physical health outcomes.	<ul><li>Racism was associated with poorer mental health, physical health, and general health.</li><li>Effect sizes of racism on mental health were stronger in cross-sectional compared with longitudinal data and in non-representative samples compared with representative samples.</li><li>Age, sex, birthplace, and education level did not moderate the effects of racism on health.</li><li>Ethnicity significantly moderated the effect of racism on negative mental health and physical health.</li><li>The association between racism and negative mental health was significantly stronger for Asian American and Latino(a) American participants compared with African American participants.</li><li>The association between racism and physical health was significantly stronger for Latino(a) American participants compared with African American participants.</li></ul>	<ul><li>Racism can occur at multiple levels, including internalized, interpersonal, and systemic.</li><li>Racism persists as a cause of exclusion, conflict and disadvantage on a global scale, and racism is increasing in many national contexts.</li><li>Racism can impact health via several recognized pathways.</li><li>Stronger association between racism and mental health outcomes, compared with physical health.</li><li>Racism has long-term effects on health that remain significant despite attenuation over time.</li></ul>

Kershaw KN et al. (2016)[52]	To identify relationships between segregation of Blacks, Hispanics/Latinos, and Asians and obesity and diabetes and to identify knowledge gaps on whether and how segregation influences these conditions.	• Eight studies of adults examined residential segregation and BMI/obesity. • Little overlap in geographic scale of segregation (metropolitan versus neighborhood), race/ethnicity of the population, and cut points used to assess segregation. • Associations between neighborhood-level segregation and BMI/obesity were largely null. • Relation between metropolitan area-level segregation and obesity revealed the complex relationship it has with health, found heterogeneity in the impact of segregation on obesity by gender, ethnicity, and racial identity among Hispanics. • No association between racial/ethnic residential segregation and diabetes prevalence, but higher segregation of Blacks was related to higher diabetes mortality.	• Cross-sectional studies, and even most longitudinal studies, cannot adequately capture the hypothesized impact of segregation on health. • Current study models could not account socioeconomic attainment, which begins in childhood and impacts adult levels. • Given the different historical context of segregation among Asians and Hispanics/Latinos, the challenge of defining segregation adequately for these groups remain unsolved. • Alternative modeling strategies and study designs will need to be applied to improve understanding of the role of segregation in health.

continued

Table 1.2 *continued*

Author/year	Study objectives	Key findings	Themes
Landrine H et al. (2017)[53]	To answer the following five questions: 1) Does racial residential segregation contribute to cancer incidence, mortality, survival, risk, screening, and/or stage at diagnosis? 2) What measures of segregation are used? 3) What types of cancers are examined? 4) Do studies of cancer patients focus on a single state or on multiple states? 5) What are the modera-tors/mediators of segregation's role in cancer?	• Segregation contributed significantly to cancer and racial cancer disparities in 70% of analyses, even after controlling for socioeconomic status and health insurance. • Residing in segregated African American areas was associated with higher odds of later-stage diagnosis of breast and lung cancers, higher mortality rates and lower survival rates from breast and lung cancers, and higher cumulative cancer risks associated with exposure to ambient air toxics. • Most (10 of 13) cancer registry studies did not test any of myriad potential mediators. • Eight of 20 analyses used percent African American (an invalid measure) as the measure of segregation and found effects in 62% of analyses. • 60% of analyses used the isolation index or the dissimilarity index (both valid measures of segregation), and significant segregation effects were found in 75% of analyses that used these measures. However, 40% of analyses used percent African American in an area as the measure of segregation despite evidence that its validity is dubious at best.	• Although there are valid measures of segregation, they are not always used in racial disparity studies. • More studies should use well-known and valid measures of segregation (concentration, clustering, centralization, hypersegregation). • More studies should include major cancers in study of residential segregation and cancer incidence, mortality, survival, risk, screening, and/or stage at diagnosis. • Use cancer data by state, which may find that the most robust segregation measure varies by state • Studies should assess segregation at the census level instead of higher levels. • Studies should examine the health-behavior and neighborhood variables that may mediate the segregation effect.

| Groos M et al. (2018)[43] | To review the various empirical measures used by researchers for quantifying structural racism and its effects on health. | • Structural racism was generally defined as (1) residential housing patterns, (2) perceptions of structural racism in social institutions broadly, (3) SES, (4) criminal justice, (5) immigration/border enforcement, (6) political participation, (7) workplace.
• Majority of studies looked at Black-white racial comparisons, two studies considered Latino (immigration/border enforcement policies), and one study considered Chinese-Americans (home mortgage discrimination). | • Focuses on studies measuring structural, institutional racism.
• Considers structural racism as fundamental cause of health inequities.
• Many quantitative, if occasionally abstract, ways to examine structural racism exist.
• Multiple studies used self-report to quantify subjects' perception of racism.
• Generally objective measures (e.g., blood pressure) were used to quantify health outcomes.
• Few studies defined structural racism and direct effect on health. |

continued

Table 1.2 *continued*

Author/year	Study objectives	Key findings	Themes
Heard-Garris NJ et al. (2018)[54]	To identify definitions of vicarious racism used in the literature, instruments used to measure racism, and vicarious racism exposure pathways that may influence child health.	• Most studies were published after 2011 in urban areas in the US, employed longitudinal designs, and focused on African American populations. Socioemotional and mental health outcomes were most commonly reported with statistically significant associations with vicarious racism. • No standard definition of vicarious racism used. • Of the 30 total studies reviewed, 73 health outcomes were reported, and of these, 38 (52%) were statistically significantly associated with indirectly experienced racism and a child health outcome. • 48% of all health outcomes assessed had no statistically significant relationship with the child health outcome studied. • Within the pre-birth studies, maternal perceived racial discrimination was found to be negatively associated with birthweight and positively associated with preterm birth. • 48% of the post-birth studies reported statistically significant relationships between vicarious racism and child health. • Almost half of the studies reported statistically significant mediators or moderators between racism and the child health outcomes examined.	• Two different exposure pathways presented (1) pre-birth pathway, classified as prenatal exposure to maternal racial discrimination, (2) post-birth pathway, further divided into two sub-pathways: (2a) caregiver exposure pathway, where children are exposed to vicarious racism through their caregivers' direct racial discrimination experiences, (2b) the non-caregiver exposure pathway, which includes racism experienced through other sources. • Lack of standard definition of vicarious racism or consensus on how best to measure exposure underscores critical need to focus on conceptualization and measurement of this type of racism exposure. • The relationship between vicarious racism and child health requires more study, as a child's exposure to racism may occur through caregivers, peers, media, and the internet.

| Smith BP et al. (2018)[55] | To understand the relationship between urban neighborhood and residential factors and breast cancer incidence and prognosis in African American women | • African American women living in low SES have greater odds of late-stage breast cancer diagnosis and mortality.
• African American women living in segregated areas (higher percentage of Blacks) have higher odds of late stage diagnosis and mortality compared to White and Hispanic women living in less segregated areas (lower percentage of Blacks).
• Late-stage diagnosis was significantly higher in areas with poor mammography access and areas with higher Black residential segregation.
• Residential pollution did not affect breast cancer risk in African American women. | • Qualitative synthesis of major neighborhood and residential factors of breast cancer outcomes in African American women.
• Lack of carefully designed studies specifically focusing on breast cancer disparities in African American women due to urban residential and neighborhood factors. |

continued

Table 1.2 *continued*

Author/year	Study objectives	Key findings	Themes
Castle B et al. (2019)[56]	To analyze the extent to which public health currently addresses systemic racism against Black Americans in the published literature.	<ul><li>Some articles discussed potential approaches to studying and addressing systemic racism in public health, including application of anti-racist praxis, critical race theory, and intersectionality.</li><li>Many papers acknowledge impact of racial residential segregation but do not emphasize its systemic characteristics; many papers fail to explicitly use the term "systemic racism."</li><li>Few articles (7) address health policy and its relationship with health disparities and systemic racism; the papers that did focus on policy discussed the importance of macro-level structural changes to improve lives of Black people and other people of color.</li><li>Articles discussing systemic racism's impact on health looked to influence of news topics on health agendas, how racial inequity in the justice system translates to health disparities for minorities, and the relationship between majority white public health leadership and sparsity of research in racism.</li></ul>	<ul><li>Focuses on systemic, structural, institutional racism.</li><li>Four major themes emerged during the review of articles: (1) approaches to address systemic racism, (2) the impact of residential and racial segregation on health outcomes, (3) policy implications for reducing health inequities, (4) systemic racism's impact on health outcomes.</li><li>Many articles did not use the term "racism" or "structural racism"; instead, they used terms such as "discrimination," "stigma," and "bias."</li><li>For studies recommending individual-level interventions for better health outcomes, many of the behavioral recommendations are not conducive to environments that are plagued with the effects of systemic racism.</li><li>While there is growing support for systemic racism as a root cause of health outcomes, there are few acknowledgments of the implications of systemic racism or interventions/ policies that address this root cause.</li><li>Must examine intersection of different forms of systemic discrimination.</li></ul>

Forde AT et al. (2019)[57]	To summarize the literature empirically testing the weathering hypothesis, assess the quality of the evidence regarding weathering as a determinant of racial disparities in health, and evaluate the threats to validity of existing studies.	• Most studies (78%) used a cross-sectional design and the remaining 22% of studies used a cohort design. • Evidence for weathering was observed in studies on birth outcomes, physical health, and self-reported health. • 14 out of 20 tests showed weathering was more likely to be observed in the socioeconomically disadvantaged group than the socioeconomically advantaged group. • Studies on telomere length, chronic stress, inflammation, and epigenetics also found support for weathering.	• Weathering is the result of chronic exposure to social and economic disadvantage that leads to the acceleration of normal aging and earlier onset of unfavorable physical health conditions among disadvantaged persons of similar age. • The weathering hypothesis has contributed significantly to literature on racial disparities in birth outcomes. • Lack of studies examining weathering within the Hispanic population by race or within the Black population by nativity status makes this an important focus for future research on weathering. • Cross-sectional studies lack advantage of longitudinal studies beginning early in the life course in characterizing how disadvantage and health coevolve over the life course.

continued

Table 1.2 *continued*

Author/year	Study objectives	Key findings	Themes
Yang TC et al. (2020)[58]	To investigate the relationships between racial/ethnic segregation and health and evaluate the extent to which racial/ethnic segregation may account for health disparities.	• The majority of studies (56 out of 66) reported that segregation adversely affects health outcomes and/or widens racial/ethnic health disparities, particularly between Blacks and Whites. • Five studies found that segregation improves health outcomes among Blacks or narrows racial/ethnic health disparities. • Among Hispanics, a protective effect of segregation has been found on coronary heart disease risk, physical disability, the disparities in early diagnosis of breast cancer, obesity, self-rated health, mental distress, and maternal smoking. • Four of the seven studies that explicitly measured white/Asian segregation found that Asians benefited from high segregation in terms of low risk of having a low-birth-weight baby and smoking during pregnancy, low odds of late-stage breast cancer diagnosis and early-stage breast cancer surgery, and low sodium-potassium ratio. • 13 studies did not find a significant relationship between racial/ethnic segregation and health disparities.	• Future research should explore other racial/ethnic segregation dimensions, particularly beyond exposure and evenness; studies should also compare whether different approaches to measuring neighborhood segregation change the findings. • The spatial scales for segregation measures need to be clarified. • The effect of segregation between Whites and non-Black minorities, particularly Hispanics and Asians, need to be studied more. • The scope of health outcomes should be further expanded to include mental health, substance use, and use of mental health care. • Longitudinal research design needed to answer the question whether segregation carries a long-term effect on health.

| Alson et al. (2021)[59] | To identify quantitative measures of systemic racism salient across reproductive health outcomes. | • For civil rights laws and legal racial discrimination, measures include cohort construction around passage of 1964 Civil Rights Act, Jim Crow designation, timing/geography of legislation.
• For residential/housing discrimination, measures include Index of Concentration at the Extremes, Area Deprivation Index, Redlining Index, Racial Bias in Mortgage Lending Index.
• For police violence, measures include Survey of Police-Public Encounters data, estimated rates of police killings by geography, police violence items in contextualized stress measure.
• For mass incarceration, there are no established measures but some are suggested.
• A multidimensional measure of structural racism measures state-level differences in the Black–White relative proportions of four domains: (1) political participation, (2) employment and job status, (3) educational attainment, (4) judicial treatment. | • Guided by three theoretical schools of thought: (1) Ecosocial Theory, (2) Fundamental Cause Theory, (3) Public Health Critical Race Praxis.
• Four domains of systemic racism affecting reproductive health: (1) civil rights laws and legal racial discrimination, (2) residential segregation and housing discrimination, (3) police violence, (4) mass incarceration.
• Employing multidimensional measures of structural racism may help understand interlocking and compounding harms that can be obscured by single domain measures.
• Research cannot only focus on individual-level racism, systemic racism requires empirical attention to deconstruct its contributions to racial inequities in reproductive health.
• Intervening in a single domain of structural racism without consideration of the greater whole and its dynamic nature will not effectively contribute to reduction in racial inequities. |

continued

Table 1.2 *continued*

Author/year	Study objectives	Key findings	Themes
Rudes et al. (2021)[60]	To address the question: "Is belonging to a minority group a risk factor for suicidality among young people in developed countries?"	• 20 studies out of 23 studies suggested a positive relationship between suicidality and young people belonging to a minority group in developed countries. • Acculturation, interpreted as the assimilation of the dominant culture with the loss of values from one's cultural background, is the main suicide risk factor. • Further suicide risks include historical loss, ancestry discrimination, and maternal discrimination. • 16 out of 23 studies demonstrated links between racial/ethnic discrimination and depressive symptoms.	• Considers studies measuring specific and broader forms of racism. • Racism can lead to suicidal ideation and suicidal attempts among minority groups, with a strong association between acculturation and suicidality. • Studying factors and suicidal behaviors related to racism in other countries, especially where migration is growing, may help understand risk better. • Mental health problems affect 1 in every 10 young people, and 70% of young people with a psychological problem have not had appropriate interventions. • Suicide prevention is especially critical in schools and in community settings, where racism is relevant and negatively affects the mental health of young people.

Mapping the Literature on Structural Racism and Racial/Ethnic Health Inequities

Several themes emerged from the retrieved studies. First, there was an increase in the number of relevant publications in 2020 and 2021 in the wake of COVID-19 and renewed social protest against racism in the United States. Second, the quantity and quality of evidence linking structural racism and health outcomes varies substantially depending on the pathway examined through which structural racism may influence health. While there is ample evidence linking disparities in the built environment with poor health outcomes among racial/ethnic minority groups—and to a lesser extent the population in general—research linking disparities in education, employment, and the judicial system to racial and ethnic inequities in health outcomes is lacking.

Third, the majority of retrieved research is descriptive, with only a few studies assessing experimental evidence or interventions to address structural racism with a goal of tackling health inequities.

Fourth, evidence is primarily based on cross-sectional, not longitudinal, data. This can affect the ability to assess temporality and can potentially partially explain the lack of interventions because the evidence base is ill-defined. Fifth, studies mostly compared the health outcomes of Black and White Americans, but empirical evidence on structural racism and the health of Native Americans and Asian Americans is lacking. Further, there was little differentiation between race and ethnicity or the experiences of communities that overlap in their racial and ethnic groups.

Sixth, among the health outcomes assessed, there is limited research that unpacks how different structural racism forces shape disparities in maternal mortality, unintentional accidents and injuries, mental health, and asthma. Beyond these overall themes, we organize the retrieved literature according to the different pathways by which structural racism can shape racial/ethnic health inequities in the United States.

Education and Health Inequities

The literature on the links between racial and ethnic disparities in education and health inequities emerged from a relatively small number of articles. Overall, the existing literature focused on educational attainment and years of school as exposures, while a few analyses assessed inter-generational educational mobility, school desegregation, and educational experiences.

The paucity of research in this area highlights the need to further investigate the links between educational disparities and health. The common research practice of subsuming education as one among the many socioeconomic factors represented by a single composite indicator is, in many cases, a hindrance to estimating the potential effect of racial and ethnic inequities in education on health outcomes.

Employment and Financial Strain, and Health Inequities

Overall, we identified a small number of articles that focused on employment and financial strain. Research on structural racism in job security and health outcomes, particularly mental health, is limited. Moreover, there is lack of research on growing sectors, such as gig economy jobs, childcare, and long-term care workers and health.

COVID-19 put the spotlight on existing racial/ethnic differences in health vulnerabilities directly linked to employment opportunities. Analyses during the pandemic demonstrated that, generally, racial/ethnic minority groups were more likely to work in occupations and sectors that exposed them to unique hazards compared to their White counterparts. Research also examined how racial/ethnic minority groups had less agency in practicing preventive health behaviors. A few analyses also highlighted emerging research that focused both on the effects of employment and economic security on the studied persons and on their entire household.

Healthcare Access and Quality, and Health Inequities

There is a growing literature that demonstrates how inequities in healthcare can shape racial/ethnic health inequities, particularly cancer-related outcomes. There exists a more robust literature, including experimental or interventional studies, on inequities in access and quality of health compared to the other pathways through which structural racism affects health. This showcases a growing awareness of the importance of engaging the healthcare system to tackle racial and ethnic health disparities.

However, the retrieved literature also highlighted two gaps in scholarship on inequities in the healthcare systems when it comes to health outcomes studied. First, research related to health outcomes—such as mental health, asthma, maternal deaths, and unintentional injuries—in relation to racial and ethnic disparities in healthcare is scarce. Second, studies that focused on cancer-related outcomes largely focused on colorectal and breast cancers.

The Built Environment and Health Inequities

Three main exposure themes emerged from articles focused on the built environment and health inequities: neighborhood conditions, residential segregation, and historical practices of structural racism. The majority of studies examined racial/ethnic inequities in neighborhood conditions—including neighborhood poverty, education, urbanicity, public housing, housing density, economic deprivation, and access to various built environment infrastructure such as grocery stores. The studies that examined residential segregation often used zip codes, residential zoning, and ethnic enclaves for analyses. Finally, a body of work examined historically racist practices, included redlining, mortgage practices, and lending bias. Various indexes of measurements were used in studies on the built environment and health inequities, including the neighborhood deprivation index, the social vulnerability index, and the dissimilarity index.

The links between structural racism and the built environment were particularly evident in comparisons between Black and White persons, in which Black individuals overwhelmingly had a greater burden of poor health, including cancers, HIV/AIDS, asthma, obesity, life expectancy, cardiovascular diseases, diabetes, mental health, diabetes, and, more recently, COVID-19.

The ample research in this area highlights the need to move from research describing disparities in the built environment and health inequities to focusing on either specific mechanisms or interventions that address such disparities. Moreover, there is a need to conduct research on the emerging phenomenon of gentrification and its potential impact on health inequities.

The Judicial System and Health Inequities

There is a relative shortage of peer-reviewed literature that assesses the links between judicial system disparities and health inequities. The lack of relevant articles spotlights the need for more research in this area. The included studies demonstrate preliminary insights that racial disparities in incarceration rates and age of incarceration are linked to inequities in health outcomes. These studies mostly focus on Black Americans and mental health outcomes.

However, it was clear that the existing literature often does not explicitly connect structural racism and negative health outcomes for incarcerated communities. In most cases, the connection is implied. Further, there were limited analyses examining the relationships between structural racism in incarceration and chronic illnesses, such as cardiovascular disease and cancer.

Interventional Studies and Health Inequities

Beyond understanding the landscape of the peer-reviewed literature on structural racism and health inequities, we aimed to document the presence and effectiveness of existing efforts to tackle structural racism with the goal of improving health outcomes in the United States. Such studies can provide insights on potential actionable areas to invest in and scale. Across the retrieved literature, 19 studies analyzed interventions aimed to address the effects of structural racism on health, 15 of which were published in the last three years, showing a growing interest in establishing empirical evidence for action. Fifteen of the studies assessed interventions directly related to healthcare access and quality disparities. Two studies focused on addressing inequities in the educational system, and the remaining two focused on employment and the built environment each (Table 1.3).

The majority of the interventional analyses that examined interventions related to healthcare access and quality assessed the effects of legislation on health outcomes, including the ACA, Medicaid expansion and/or Medicare expansion,[18-24] the Mental Health Parity and Addictions Equality Act,[25,26] and mandated physician-patient communication policy.[27] The other five studies examined integrated patient navigation systems,[28] expansion of COVID-19 testing facilities,[29] collaborative care management,[30] and

Table 1.3 Summary of relevant studies that assessed interventions

Structural racism pathway	Outcome	Study overview	Key findings
Education/ desegregation	Mental health/executive function	Peterson et al. analyzed a survey of aged 50+ included in the Healthy Aging in African Americans (STAR) cohort study in 2018–19.[33]	Compared to children who did not move to integrated school, children who moved to integrated school had better executive function and memory.
Education/state school policies	Overall health/late-life physical and mental health	Willa et al. tested whether improvements in quantity and quality of education between 1908 and 1962 were associated with improved overall perceived physical and mental health in Reasons for Geographic and Racial Differences in Stroke (REGARDS) cohort.[34]	State-based school quality and quantity policies have a causal effect on improved late-life mental and physical health, especially for older Black adults.
Employment/ workplace safety measures	COVID infection rate	Herstein et al. studied 13 Nebraska meat processing facilities where COVID-19 was diagnosed in 5002 workers out of about 26,000 between April 1–July 31, 2020. They also examined effect of initiating both universal masking and physical barrier interventions at meat processing facilities during the COVID-19 pandemic.[35]	After initiating both universal masking and physical barrier interventions, 8/13 facilities showed a statistically significant reduction in COVID-19 incidence in within 10 days. Although 67% of confirmed cases were among workers of Hispanic or Latino ethnicity, they constituted 78% of ICU admissions and 86% of deaths, indicating a higher burden of poor outcomes among this group. The intervention therefore helped to improve outcomes in general, and particularly for minorities.

continued

Table 1.3 *continued*

Structural racism pathway	Outcome	Study overview	Key findings
Housing/residential segregation	cardiovascular risk	D'Agostino et al. examined data from multisite park-based afterschool physical activity program, Fit2Play, in Miami, FL to test association between change in residential segregation and cardiovascular health outcomes across race/ethnicity and gender for youth. They also tested whether minority youth participating at park sites with lower residential segregation relative to their home neighborhood would have greater improvements in cardiovascular health compared with those at park sites with the same or higher levels of residential segregation.[36]	The study found statistically significant improvements in cardiovascular health including obesity (BMI), skinfold thicknesses, blood pressure, and 400m run time were found for youth who attended the program in a less segregated area compared with their home area. Non-Hispanic Black girls showed the greatest cardiovascular health improvements.
Healthcare/coverage expansion	Breast cancer	Biggers et al. examined role of Medicare subsidies in reducing Black–White disparities in breast cancer outcomes attributable to the high cost of breast cancer adjuvant hormonal (endocrine) therapy. The authors used Medicare D enrollees' data and examined a nationwide cohort of women 65+ with a breast cancer operation between 2006 and 2007. Non-adherence and no-claims were analyzed, and survival analysis was conducted, after adjusting for major factors that may affect the outcome.[22]	The analysis showed that unsubsidized women were 60% to 200% more likely to discontinue hormonal therapy in the first 35 months compared with the recipients of the same race or ethnicity. The study found that prescription subsidy was associated with substantially improved persistence to breast cancer hormonal therapy among all races. This study shows that policy interventions can improve equity in cancer outcomes.

| Healthcare/coverage expansion | Breast cancer | Sempirini et al. evaluated the effect of Medicaid expansion on Black/White breast cancer mortality disparities found that the Medicaid expansion led to increase in disparity between Black and White women and more so in younger age groups (and ages 45 to 49, 50 to 54). The authors used state level cancer mortality data from CDC and compared across states—first between all expanding states and all nonexpanding states, then between all expanding states and nonexpanding states that voted to expand but did not by January 2014. They also used difference in difference method and adjusted for other factors that might affect the result.[19] | Medicaid expansion led to increase in disparity between Black and White women and more so in younger age groups (45–49, 50–54).

The study concluded that states cannot solely rely on access to insurance to address disparities in cancer and that low-quality health systems may need to be examined as well.

One caveat with the analysis is the ecological nature of data, which means the result may be different when we analyze the data at the patient level rather than at a state level. |

continued

Table 1.3 *continued*

Structural racism pathway	Outcome	Study overview	Key findings
Healthcare/coverage expansion	Colorectal cancer	Yasmin et al. examined the effect of Medicaid expansion on colorectal cancer screening rates. They used the difference in difference method, and analyzed Behavior Risk Factor Surveillance System data, nationally representative health-related telephone survey data, from 2012 to 2016.[18]	Colorectal cancer screening decreased incidence and improves survival, but minorities have lower screening rates. The study showed that overall screening in expansion states increased compared with no expansion states. For Black respondents, there was a significant increase in early expansion states, but no change in late expansion states. The study also found that there was no significant change for Hispanic respondents in early or 2014 expansion states. But as the study notes, the populations from early expansion, 2014/Medicaid expansion, and no expansion states, are notably different, with a higher proportion of low-income respondents in no expansion states and more Black respondents in no expansion states compared to more Hispanics in early expansion states. The issue with ecological analysis holds true with this study, and the result may be different when we analyze the data on insurance status at the patient level rather than at a state level.

| Healthcare/coverage expansion | Colorectal cancer | Powell et al. examined the effect of ACA in North Carolina, which did not expand Medicaid. The authors used a simulation model to estimate the impact of ACA (increasing insurance through health exchanges alone or with Medicaid expansion) on screening, stage-specific incidence, and deaths related to colorectal cancer. They also analyzed the impact on the economic costs among African American and White males who were age-eligible for screening (between ages 50 and 75) during the study period.[20] | The simulation showed that Medicaid expansion improved colon cancer outcomes overall, though the impact was more substantial among African Americans.

Medicaid expansion would prevent between 7.1 to 25.5 cases per 100,000 CRC cases among African Americans and between 4.1 to 16.4 among White males.

The study suggests that policies improving healthcare coverage could have a cost-saving impact while reducing cancer disparities. The study is limited by the design. |
| Healthcare/coverage expansion | Colorectal cancer | Mobley et al. examined Medicare modernization implemented in 2006 to increase managed care options for seniors and free up budgets for Medicare fee-for-service (FFS) enrollees, making copayments for colorectal cancer (CRC) screenings possible. The authors assessed the data on Medicare FFS enrollees aged 65+ each year during 2001–2005, or 2006–2009, to see what happened to the screening rates and what factors affected the changes. They accounted for other factors that may affect the result.[21] | The study cited three policy changes that occurred after 2006 and state-specific CRC interventions aimed at minorities over the decade as possible reasons responsible for the observed improvements: (1) Medicare subsidies to provide prescription drug coverage, which eased budgets for seniors, (2) elimination of the out-of-pocket copay for CRC screening, (3) an external factor which is inclusion of CRC screening by endoscopy as part of the gold standard by the scientific community.

The study found an increase of more than 850,000 endoscopic procedures per year.

The authors concluded that disparities in the utilization of CRC screening declined over time in many states. |

continued

Table 1.3 *continued*

Structural racism pathway	Outcome	Study overview	Key findings
Healthcare/coverage expansion	Colorectal cancer	Jayakrishnan et al. used the National Cancer Database (NCDB) to examine the changes in enrollment to primary therapies for colorectal cancer following ACA and analyzed the impact on outcomes. They used data between 2004 and 2015 and calculated Time to initiation (time in days from the date of diagnosis of cancer to earliest date of initiation of first line cancer directed therapy) before and after ACA using 2001 as a cut-off.[24]	The data of more than 130,000 late-stage colorectal cancer patients showed that the difference between races on colon cancer treatment enrollment became insignificant post-ACA. For rectal cancer, the enrollment rates in fact improved for Black persons more than White persons post-ACA. However, the poorer mortality rate among Blacks continued even after ACA.
Healthcare/coverage expansion	HIV testing	Gai et al. examined association between ACA and HIV testing and risk behavior using data from the 2010 to 2017 the Behavioral Risk Factor Surveillance System. They used the difference in differences method for their analysis.[23]	The study showed that Medicaid expansion promoted HIV testing without increasing HIV risk behavior. The study found that, compared with non-expansion states, expansion states had a 3.22% increase in HIV tests. Though the impacts on HIV tests were larger for non-Hispanic Blacks, the disparities persisted. The study concluded that non-expansion states, mostly in the South, missed an opportunity and could face serious health and financial consequences as a result.

| Healthcare/New York law on mandatory communications | postmastectomy breast reconstruction (PBR) | The study by Mahoudi et al. examined the effect of 2011 State of New York law in reducing racial/ethnic disparities in immediate PBR (IPBR). The law mandated that physicians communicate about reconstructive surgery with patients undergoing mastectomy. This is a relevant legislative intervention for postmastectomy breast reconstruction (PBR), as wide disparities in the use of PBR exist despite its demonstrated benefits.[27] | By examining more than 42,000 women, including 19,364 from New York (experiment group) and 22,982 from California (comparison group), and using the difference-in-differences methods, the researchers showed that the law led to the reduction in disparities in IPBR between Hispanic and white patients by 9% and between other minorities and white patients by 13%. The study also showed that the gap in disparity between Whites and African Americans persisted. The authors conclude that the lack of patient trust or effective physician-patient communication may be the potential cause for the reduced effect of mandatory communication for some subpopulations, including African American individuals. |

continued

Table 1.3 *continued*

Structural racism pathway	Outcome	Study overview	Key findings
Healthcare/mental health parity and addictions equality act (MHPAEA)	Depression	Goldberg et al. examined the depression treatment choice in primary care facilities. They analyzed 2007–2012 National Ambulatory Medical Care Survey, representing 162 million depressed patients in the US.[26]	Overall Non-Hispanic Blacks and Hispanics received treatment at the lowest rates (71.3% and 75.4%, respectively). The study found that treatment was significantly more likely to be provided after the MHPAEA. Patients were less likely to be prescribed only medication than only psychotherapy after the MHPAEA. The authors note that the persisting differences may be accounted for by racial stereotypes or by stigma against seeking mental health care that occur in minority communities.
Healthcare/mental health parity and addictions equality act (MHPAEA)	Alcohol treatment access	Mulia et al. analyzed data from SAMHSA'S Treatment Episode Data Set (TEDS) from 1999 to 2013, to assess changes in alcohol treatment admission rates across states.[25]	The study found a significantly greater increase in treatment rates in states that required health insurance plans to cover alcohol treatment. This was seen overall and in all three racial/ethnic groups (increasing by 25% in Whites, 26% in Blacks, and 42% in Hispanics above the expected treatment rate for these groups). Post-MHPAEA, the alcohol treatment admissions rate in these states rose to the level of states with the strongest pre-existing parity laws. However, the changes were of roughly similar magnitude in Whites, Blacks, and Hispanics.

| Healthcare/patient navigation system | Breast cancer screening | Henderson et al. assessed the Mile Square Accessible Mammogram Outreach and Engagement (Mi-MAMO) using an implementation science framework. The Mile Square Health Centers (MSHC) that has 12 federally qualified health centers implemented the program with a goal to support under resourced women to mitigate multilevel barriers to mammography screening by providing free breast cancer screening and diagnostic services.[28] | The early results indicate that 95.5% of those who use the services were racial/ethnic minorities. The program is being expanded to include large-scale implementation across all MSHC primary care sites and two community hospitals outside the university health system for wider system-level adoption. |
| Healthcare/ decentralized care | COVID Testing rate | Hernandez et al. analyzed the effectiveness of the New Orleans Health Department (NOHD) partnership with a local healthcare network (LCMC) to deploy mobile testing sites throughout the city in early 2020 in improving testing rates.[29] | The study analyzed testing data recorded for 9,721 patients at 20 sites during May–June 2020

Used maps to show the changes in testing coverage for minority neighborhoods and calculated the actual distance covered by individuals.

The study concluded that walk-up sites significantly increased testing availability in New Orleans, and specifically in minority neighborhoods. Both African Americans and Asians were more likely (14.7% and 53.0%) to be tested at the nearest walk-up site. Hispanics, however, were not associated with increased proximity to and use of nearest sites. |

continued

Table 1.3 *continued*

Structural racism pathway	Outcome	Study overview	Key findings
Healthcare/ decentralized care	Cancer survival	Ailawadhi et al. examined the impact of access to designated cancer centers on multiple myeloma (MM) treatment and outcome.[32] The National Cancer Act 1971 formalized the establishment of designated cancer centers to improve quality and efficiency of cancer care. They analyzed cancer registry (Surveillance, Epidemiology, and End Results, SEER) database for patients diagnosed with myeloma between 1973 and 2011.	The study analyzed more than 70,000 patients and found that the proportion of white patients with access to ≥ 2 national centers or 1 network centers progressively declined over time (from 55.95% to 48.4%), whereas access for Asians (from 5.8% to 9%) and Hispanics (from 18.4% to 23.8%) increased. However, for African Americans there was marginal decrease in access to national center and marginal increase in access to network centers. Survival improvement was seen in patients with access to ≥ 1 national center versus none, and no survival improvement was seen in patients with access to 1 national center. The study concluded that survival improvement was not observed among nonwhites despite potential access to ≥ 2 national centers. This may reflect referral patterns from community practitioners, insurance coverage and participation, a lack of awareness, or patient preference driven by sociocultural beliefs advocating care in a smaller setting rather than larger care centers.

| Healthcare/ decentralized care | Same-day angioplasty | Hsia et al. used inpatient data of around 140,000 myocardial infarction patients between 2006 and 2015, from the California Office of Statewide Health Planning and Development, and regionalized care arrangement information from all 33 local EMS agencies and looked at three outcomes access to hospitals with angioplasty facility to open blocked arteries of heart, treatment, and mortality.[31] | The study found a 6.3% increase in access to hospitals for residents in nonminority communities after they were exposed to regionalization, while patients in a minority community had a smaller improvement (1.8 percentage points). After regionalization, White individuals in nonminority communities experienced a 5.4% (statistically significant) increase in the probability of receiving same-day angioplasty, but Black or Hispanic patients living in minority communities did not accrue any benefit. For mortality, White residents of nonminority communities experienced improvements in 30-day, 90-day, and 1-year mortality, while none of these improvements in mortality were experienced by other groups. One reason that authors cited for this difference is that patients with heart attack from minority communities use EMS less often than those from nonminority communities. A larger reason may also be that the practice in hospitals or regions that serve patients in minority communities are systemically different from those that serve nonminority communities. |

continued

Table 1.3 *continued*

Structural racism pathway	Outcome	Study overview	Key findings
Healthcare/ collaborative care for mental illness	Depression	Angstman et al. tested whether use of collaborative care management (CCM) in treating depressed primary care patients would decrease racial disparities in clinical outcomes.[30] The team reviewed the medical chart of 3,588 (51.2%) patients who received usual care and 3,422 (48.8%) patients who were enrolled in CCM.	The data showed that minority patients enrolled in CCM were more likely to be participating in depression care at 6 months than minority patients in UC (61.9% vs. 14.4%). The difference remained significant even after adjusting for other relevant factors. Minority patients in CCM had significantly improved outcomes with 50.3% reaching remission (vs. 10.2% in normal care). The study concluded that collaborative care significantly reduces disparities for outcomes of compliance, remission, or persistence of depressive symptoms for minority patients with depression

decentralization of care.[31,32] Six studies looked at cancer as an outcome, and one looked into HIV testing rates. Four of these studies showed that the health outcomes of racial and ethnic minority groups improved, two showed mixed results, and one study found that the health outcomes of racial/ethnic minority groups worsened following the intervention. The gap in health outcomes between racial and ethnic groups decreased only in one study among the four studies that showed that outcomes improved for minority groups, while two reported mixed results and one study did not report on the gap.

Both analyses evaluating interventions in the educational system were longitudinal in nature, which gives strength to the evidence generated. Both studies showed that outcomes improved for racial/ethnic minority groups.[33,34] The study that assessed an employment intervention looked at COVID-19 incidence following the initiation of public health measures and found that health outcomes improved in general, and particularly for racial/ethnic minority groups.[35] The study on the built environment described a natural experiment that analyzed the association between changes in residential segregation and cardiovascular health outcomes. The study found that the health outcomes of racial/ethnic minority groups improved following the implementation of the intervention.[36]

Learning from the Literature: A Path Forward

The findings documented in this chapter can provide a roadmap for action for institutions concerned with tackling racial and ethnic racial health inequities in the United States. We propose a strategy—which can be taken as a whole or in part to complement other necessary courses of action—based on the findings that emerged from our review of the literature as well as from our experience in the field and in conversation with scholars concerned with structural racism.

As with any proposed strategy, these recommendations should be read with a clear understanding of the limitations of the efforts that led to them. In particular, we have applied a specific, rigorous, academic lens to our review of the literature, but we are also aware that other efforts may lead to different recommendations. Further, scientific inquiry does not exist in a vacuum, and it is important to note that the questions being answered in this chapter emerge from a system that is itself shaped by structural racism.

With those caveats articulated, we propose a four-part strategy, which can be adopted by institutions if they were to commit to efforts to limit the influence of structural racism on health in the United States. While we articulate 18 recommendations, we do not present them in order of importance but rather organize them as part of a comprehensive strategy. We do not intend recommendation 1 to be seen as more important than recommendation 18.

Advocate

Institutions can invest in advocating for structural changes in sectors where the evidence shows that improvement could potentially lead to narrowing racial and ethnic disparities in health indicators. Our recommendation in this area is largely based on the evidence from the interventions identified as efficacious in the literature, even as we note that conclusive evidence was scarce.

Recommendation One

Investment in advocacy efforts that can lead to states expanding access to healthcare, particularly through expanding insurance coverage. The literature indicates that even expansion of access to healthcare that did not directly aim to tackle disparities in health can lead to improvements in the health outcomes of minority groups, particularly in cancer-related and mental health outcomes. This shows that there should be efforts, funding, and strategic alliances to advocate for state- and city-level legislation to improve access to healthcare. In the short term, institutions can advocate for reforms in states that are reluctant to expand Medicaid.

Importantly, the literature showed that while legislation that improved healthcare access improved the health outcomes of racial and ethnic minority groups, it did not necessarily reduce the overall gap in health outcomes between different racial and ethnic groups. Addressing such gaps will likely mean investing in a larger set of interventions that extend well beyond healthcare. However, the evidence on interventions that have improved societal determinants of health and, as a result, can narrow racial/ethnic health gaps is sparse. That does not mean that advocacy on improving broader determinants of health might not indeed mitigate the effects of structural racism on health, but it does highlight that advocacy often requires an evidence base. The evidence on healthcare reflects a focus of the scholarship on healthcare, with little investment in generating impact evaluations of interventions on the broader determinants of health.

Test and Support Solutions

While the best evidence points to advocacy around expanding healthcare access as important to addressing structural racism in relation to health, there are undoubtedly many other areas where advocacy could help toward this goal. The challenge is that there is limited evidence that can point to where specific action levers can mitigate the impact of structural racism on health. This in turn points to another potential area of action—the development and testing of interventions in focused pilot projects that can be scaled up. Building on the state of the literature, we would recommend that Institutions focus on the built environment as a potential point of intervention. Evaluation efforts should also consider the potential unintended consequences of these interventions.

Recommendation Two

Fund and support analyses of existing natural experiments/interventions that could potentially mitigate racial inequities in housing and neighborhood quality. Investing in such efforts could help build the evidence base that can then point to specific actions. For example, institutions can fund specific analyses using initiatives such as Moving to Opportunity[37]—a major randomized housing mobility experiment—as well as municipal-level efforts that either improve housing for underserved communities or desegregate neighborhoods.

Recommendation Three

Establish funding for innovative pilot initiatives that aim to tackle the historical racial and ethnic inequities in housing ownership and spatial racial neighborhood segregation such as inclusionary zoning programs. These programs should both be implemented with an eye to clearly documenting success, or lack thereof, in improving the health outcomes of racial and ethnic minority groups, as well as their potential to be scaled up across the country. Institutions can also support and evaluate interventions that can address specific health determinants linked to neighborhood characteristics, such as food deserts and swamps and access to green space.

Catalyze a National Conversation

We entered this exercise with the notion that there is an abundance of literature that can point to how structural racism is linked to health. However, we ultimately found far less empirical evidence. This was possibly driven by the only relatively recent interest in the concept by the mainstream academic world and the public. We think that this represents an area of immediate need, and an opportunity for institutions to catalyze a national conversation about structural racism and its impact on health. That could then shift the Overton window, tying structural racism to health in the minds of decision-makers and the public, which would inevitably lead to a greater commitment by other entities in funding research and interventions in this area. There are a number of actors who are concerned with structural racism but not necessarily with how structural racism shapes health outcomes. This creates space for entities to focus on health, which can serve as a galvanizing force toward reducing structural racism throughout the country, affecting a whole range of other factors in time. To this end, we would recommend the following.

Recommendation Four
Develop a communication strategy to elevate visibility of the links between structural racism and health aimed at informing decision-makers, other funders, media, and, as far as possible, the general public. Such a strategy would need to involve partners who reach different audiences beyond the confines of typical communication strategies. This is a steep hill to climb, and creative approaches would be indicated.

Recommendation Five
Catalyze a broad-based national community of engagement around the idea that structural racism affects health, that we can simultaneously understand this empirically, and that we can design interventions to mitigate this historical influence. We can see such effort succeeding in elevating the visibility to one where academics, policymakers, and practitioners in both the public and private sectors all recognize the importance of addressing structural racism and health. This would be similar, for example, to how the social determinants of health used to be an area of relatively little academic and policymaking interest but several initiatives elevated the national conversation around their importance for health over the past few decades.

Invest in Research

Given the paucity of the literature on structural racism and health, we propose that investing in research, especially evaluation and translational research, is critical to advancing action to address the impact of structural racism on health in the United States. Strengthening the evidence base will then help focus institutions' advocacy and programming efforts.

Conceptual Recommendations

Recommendation Six

Fund scholarship that can lead to a more formal empirical approach to studying structural racism and that offers guidance for how data can be collected in a way that advances the field. The literature shows that there is no concrete framing around structural racism and health. This lack of formalization can then contribute to the dearth of empirical evidence and, ultimately, inaction on structural racism to improve health outcomes. Relevant research can include projects that develop methods for standardized data collection, address data gaps, and re-think racial and ethnic classifications in the United States. Institutions can also fund research on the specific pathways that potentially explain the links between structural racism and health, such as how inequities in the judicial system impact health outcomes.

Recommendation Seven

Invest in research that reports not only on whether experimental or interventional studies improve or worsen health outcomes among racial/ethnic minority groups but also if such interventions increase/reduce the gaps between different racial and ethnic groups.

Recommendation Eight

Encourage more research that takes an intergenerational and life-course approach to illustrate the effects of historical injustices on current health.

Topical Recommendations

Recommendation Nine
Prioritize research that examines the effects of structural racism on groups that include, but extend beyond Black Americans, particularly on American Indians/Native Americans.

Recommendation 10
Prioritize scholarship that focuses on health indicators about which there is a paucity of research, including maternal mortality, asthma, mental health, and unintentional injuries.

Recommendation 11
Fund research on emerging trends that will shape and be shaped by structural racism such as climate change, the gig economy, and applications of Artificial Intelligence to healthcare.

Methodological Recommendations

Recommendation 12
Require research funded to consider results stratified by race and ethnic groups instead of simply controlling for race and ethnic groups, as well as meaningfully and purposefully partner with communities when applicable.

Recommendation 13
Require funded quantitative research on structural racism to either assess multiple racial/ethnic groups to allow for inference about the relative influence of particular mechanisms on health across groups, or provide statements in their analyses when such assessment is not possible due to lack of data.

Operational Recommendations

Recommendation 14
Review existing research portfolios to ensure funding resources are aligned with the scope of the health problem borne overall and by particular racial and ethnic groups.

Recommendation 15

Invest in efforts to grow the proportion of persons from traditionally under-represented racial and ethnic groups in academia, particularly American Indians/Native Americans and Black Americans.

Recommendation 16

Counter racial and ethnic inequities in mentoring through funding mentoring opportunities for people from racial and ethnic minority groups in academia, including graduate students and postdoctoral fellows.

Recommendation 17

Create mechanisms to encourage the engagement of fields relevant, but not directly related, to public health, such as social work, economics, and sociology, in work related to structural racism and health.

Recommendation 18

Invest in translational research that uses lessons from COVID-19 about what did, and did not, widen racial and ethnic health gaps, with a particular focus on organizations that achieved success.

Acknowledgments

This chapter is based on six systematic reviews, which included several collaborators—Yvette Cozier, Collette Ncube, Elaine Nsoesie, and Julia Raifman, research analysts; Grace Robbins, Muhammed Shaffi, and Samuel Rosenberg—and student research assistants—Adaeze Okorie, Ethan Assefa, Haradeen Dhillon, Isaac Stovall, Jade Kissi, and Lintao Hu—at Boston University School of Public Health.

References

1. Bailey ZD, Feldman JM, Bassett MT. How structural racism works: Racist policies as a root cause of U.S. racial health inequities. *New England Journal of Medicine*. 2021;384(8):768–773. doi:10.1056/NEJMms2025396

2. National Center for Education Statistics. *The NCES Fast Facts Tool provides quick answers to many education questions*. Accessed November 28, 2021. https://nces.ed.gov/fastfacts.

3. Wilson V. Racial disparities in income and poverty remain largely unchanged amid strong income growth in 2019. *Economic Policy Institute*. September 16, 2020. https://www.epi.org/blog/racial-disparities-in-income-and-poverty-remain-largely-unchanged-amid-strong-income-growth-in-2019/.

4. US Census Bureau. *Quarterly residential vacancies and homeownership, second quarter 2025*. Accessed November 17, 2025. https://www.census.gov/housing/hvs/files/qtr225/Q225press.pdf.

5. Perry AM. How racial disparities in home prices reveal widespread discrimination. *Brookings*. February 24, 2021. https://www.brookings.edu/testimonies/how-racial-disparities-in-home-prices-reveal-widespread-discrimination/.

6. Desilver D, Bialik K. Blacks, Hispanics face mortgage challenges. *Pew Research Center*. January 10, 2017. https://www.pewresearch.org/fact-tank/2017/01/10/blacks-and-hispanics-face-extra-challenges-in-getting-home-loans/.

7. The Sentencing Project. *U.S. criminal justice data*. Washington, DC: The Sentencing Project. Accessed November 17, 2025. https://www.sentencingproject.org/research/us-criminal-justice-data/.

8. American Civil Liberties Union. *Mass incarceration*. Accessed November 28, 2021. https://www.aclu.org/issues/smart-justice/mass-incarceration.

9. The Sentencing Project. *Report to the United Nations on racial disparities in the U.S. criminal justice system*. Washington, DC: The Sentencing Project; 2018. https://www.sentencingproject.org/reports/report-to-the-united-nations-on-racial-disparities-in-the-u-s-criminal-justice-system/.

10. Robin C. *Health insurance coverage: Early release of estimates from the National Health Interview Survey, January–June 2020*. Washington, DC: Centers for Disease Control and Prevention; 2021. doi:10.15620/cdc:100468

11. Agency for Healthcare Research and Quality. *2019 national healthcare quality and disparities report*. US Department of Health and Human Services: Rockville, MD; 2020. https://www.ahrq.gov/research/findings/nhqrdr/nhqdr19/index.html.

12. Arias E, Betzaida TV, Ahmad F, Kochanek K. *Provisional life expectancy estimates for 2020*. Hyattsville, MD: National Center for Health Statistics; 2021. doi:10.15620/cdc:107201

13. Paradies Y, Priest N, Ben J, et al. Racism as a determinant of health: A protocol for conducting a systematic review and meta-analysis. *Systematic Reviews*. 2013;2(1):85. doi:10.1186/2046-4053-2-85

14. Pieterse AL, Todd NR, Neville HA, Carter RT. Perceived racism and mental health among Black American adults: A meta-analytic review. *Journal of Counselling Psychology*. 2012;59(1):1–9. doi:10.1037/a0026208

15. Pascoe EA, Richman LS. Perceived discrimination and health: A meta-analytic review. *Psychological Bulletin*. 2009;135(4):531–554. doi:10.1037/a0016059

16. Lee DL, Ahn, S. Racial discrimination and Asian mental health: A meta-analysis. *The Counselling Psychologist*. 2011;39(3):463–489. doi:10.1177/0011000010381791

17. Lee DL, Ahn S. Discrimination against Latina/os: A meta-analysis of individual-level resources and outcomes. *Counselling Psychologist*. 2012;40(1):28–65. doi:10.1177/0011000011403326

18. Zerhouni YA, Trinh QD, Lipsitz S, et al. Effect of Medicaid expansion on colorectal cancer screening rates. *Diseases of the Colon & Rectum*. 2019;62(1):97–103. doi:10.1097/DCR.0000000000001260

19. Semprini J, Olopade O. Evaluating the effect of Medicaid expansion on Black/White breast cancer mortality disparities: A difference-in-difference analysis. *JCO Global Oncology*. 2020;6:GO.20.00068. doi:10.1200/GO.20.00068

20. Powell W, Frerichs L, Townsley R, et al. The potential impact of the Affordable Care Act and Medicaid expansion on reducing colorectal cancer screening disparities in African American males. *PloS One*. 2020;15(1):e0226942. doi:10.1371/journal.pone.0226942

21. Mobley LR, Kuo TM, Zhou M, Rutherford Y, Meador S, Koschinsky J. What happened to disparities in CRC screening among FFS Medicare enrollees following Medicare modernization? *Journal of Racial and Ethnic Health Disparities*. 2019;6(2):273–291. doi:10.1007/s40615-018-0522-x

22. Biggers A, Shi Y, Charlson J, et al. Medicare D subsidies and racial disparities in persistence and adherence with hormonal therapy. *Journal of Clinical Oncology.* 2016;34(36):4398–4404. doi:10.1200/JCO.2016.67.3350

23. Gai Y, Marthinsen J. Medicaid expansion, HIV testing, and HIV-related risk behaviors in the United States, 2010–2017. *American Journal of Public Health.* 2019;109(10):1404–1412. doi:10.2105/AJPH.2019.305220

24. Jayakrishnan TT, Bakalov V, Chahine Z, Finley G, Monga D, Wegner RE. Impact of Affordable Care Act on the treatment and outcomes for stage-IV colorectal cancer. *Cancer Treat Research Communications.* 2020;24:100204. doi:10.1016/j.ctarc.2020.100204

25. Mulia N, Lui CK, Ye Y, Subbaraman MS, Kerr WC, Greenfield TK. U.S. alcohol treatment admissions after the Mental Health Parity and Addiction Equity Act: Do state parity laws and race/ethnicity make a difference? *Journal of Substance Abuse Treatment.* 2019;106:113–121. doi:10.1016/j.jsat.2019.08.008

26. Goldberg DM, Lin HC. Effects of the mental health parity and addictions equality act on depression treatment choice in primary care facilities. *International Journal of Psychiatry in Medicine.* 2017;52(1):34–47. doi:10.1177/0091217417703289

27. Mahmoudi E, Lu Y, Metz AK, Momoh AO, Chung KC. Association of a policy mandating physician-patient communication with racial/ethnic disparities in postmastectomy breast reconstruction. *JAMA Surgery.* 2017;152(8):775–783. doi:10.1001/jamasurg.2017.0921

28. Henderson V, Tossas-Milligan K, Martinez E, et al. Implementation of an integrated framework for a breast cancer screening and navigation program for women from under-resourced communities. *Cancer.* 2020;126 Suppl 10:2481–2493. doi:10.1002/cncr.32843

29. Hernandez JH, Karletsos D, Avegno J, Reed CH. Is Covid-19 community-level testing effective in reaching at-risk populations? Evidence from spatial analysis of New Orleans patient data at walk-up sites. *BMC Public Health.* 2021;21(1):632. doi:10.1186/s12889-021-10717-9

30. Angstman KB, Phelan S, Myszkowski MR, et al. Minority primary care patients with depression: Outcome disparities improve with collaborative care management. *Medical Care.* 2015;53(1):32–37. doi:10.1097/MLR.0000000000000280

31. Hsia RY, Krumholz H, Shen YC. Evaluation of STEMI regionalization on access, treatment, and outcomes among adults living in nonminority and minority communities. *JAMA Network Open.* 2020;3(11):e2025874. doi:10.1001/jamanetworkopen.2020.25874

32. Ailawadhi S, Advani P, Yang D, et al. Impact of access to NCI- and NCCN-designated cancer centers on outcomes for multiple myeloma patients: A SEER registry analysis. *Cancer.* 2016;122(4):618–625. doi:10.1002/cncr.29771

33. Peterson RL, George KM, Barnes LL, et al. Association of timing of school desegregation in the United States with late-life cognition in the study of healthy aging in African Americans (STAR) cohort. *JAMA Network Open.* 2021;4(10):e2129052. doi:10.1001/jamanetworkopen.2021.29052

34. Brenowitz WD, Manly JJ, Murchland AR, et al. State school policies as predictors of physical and mental health: A natural experiment in the REGARDS cohort. *American Journal of Epidemiology.* 2020;189(5):384–393. doi:10.1093/aje/kwz221

35. Herstein JJ, Degarege A, Stover D, et al. Characteristics of SARS-CoV-2 transmission among meat processing workers in Nebraska, USA, and effectiveness of risk mitigation measures. *Emerging Infectious Diseases.* 2021;27(4):1032–1038. doi:10.3201/eid2704.204800

36. D'Agostino EM, Patel HH, Ahmed Z, et al. Natural experiment examining the longitudinal association between change in residential segregation and youth cardiovascular health across race/ethnicity and gender in the USA. *Journal of Epidemiology and Community Health.* 2018;72(7):595–604. doi:10.1136/jech-2018-210592

37. National Bureau of Economic Research. *Moving to opportunity.* Accessed December 7, 2021. https://www.nber.org/programs-projects/projects-and-centers/moving-opportunity?page=1...perPage=50.

38. Bailey ZD, Krieger N, Agénor M, Graves J, Linos N, Bassett MT. Structural racism and health inequities in the USA: evidence and interventions. *The Lancet*. 2017;389 (10077):1453–1463. doi:10.1016/S0140-6736(17)30569-X

39. Gee GC, Ford CL. Structural racism and health inequities. *Du Bois Review: Social Science Research on Race*. 2011;8(1):115–132. doi:10.1017/S1742058X11000130

40. 11 terms you should know to better understand structural racism. The Aspen Institute. July 11, 2016. https://www.salisbury.edu/administration/diversity-and-inclusion/_files/anti-racism/11-terms-you-should-know-to-better-understand-structural-racism.pdf?v=2022 1105020751.

41. Krieger N. Discrimination and health inequities. *International Journal of Social Determinants of Health and Health Services*. 2014;44(4):643–710. doi:10.2190/HS.44.4.b

42. Beech P. What is environmental racism and how can we fight it? *World Economic Forum*. July 31, 2020. https://www.weforum.org/agenda/2020/07/what-is-environmental-racism-pollution-covid-systemic/.

43. Groos M, Wallace M, Hardeman R, Theall KP. Measuring inequity: A systematic review of methods used to quantify structural racism. *Journal of Health Disparities Research and Practice*. 2018;11(2):18.

44. Jim Crow law | History, facts, & examples. *Britannica*. Accessed December 11, 2021. https://www.britannica.com/event/Jim-Crow-law.

45. black code | Laws, history, & examples. *Britannica*. Accessed December 11, 2021. https://www.britannica.com/topic/black-code.

46. Reskin B. The race discrimination system. *Annual Review of Sociology*. 2012;38(1):17–35. doi:10.1146/annurev-soc-071811-145508

47. O'Brien R, Neman T, Seltzer N, Evans L, Venkataramani A. Structural racism, economic opportunity and racial health disparities: Evidence from U.S. counties. *SSM—Population Health*. 2020;11:100564. doi:10.1016/j.ssmph.2020.100564

48. Adkins-Jackson PB, Chantarat T, Bailey ZD, Ponce NA. Measuring structural racism: A guide for epidemiologists and other health researchers. *American Journal of Epidemiology*. 2021:kwab239. doi:10.1093/aje/kwab239

49. Yearby R, Watson, S, Gibson C, et al. *Governmental use of racial equity tools to address systemic racism and the social determinants of health*. Saint Louis, MO: The Institute for Healing Justice and Equity. October 19, 2021. https://ihje.org/governmental-use-of-racial-equity-tools/.

50. Corral I, Landrine H, Hall MB, Bess JJ, Mills KR, Efird JT. Residential segregation and overweight/obesity among African-American adults: A critical review. *Frontiers in Public Health*. 2015;3:169. doi:10.3389/fpubh.2015.00169

51. Kershaw KN, Albrecht SS. Racial/ethnic residential segregation and cardiovascular disease risk. *Current Cardiovascular Risk Reports*. 2015;9(3):10.

52. Kershaw KN, Pender AE. Racial/ethnic residential segregation, obesity, and diabetes mellitus. *Current Diabetes Reports*. 2016;16(11):108. doi:10.1007/s11892-016-0800-0

53. Landrine H, Corral I, Lee JGL, Efird JT, Hall MB, Bess JJ. Residential segregation and racial cancer disparities: A systematic review. *Journal of Racial & Ethnic Health Disparities*. 2017;4(6):1195–1205. doi:10.1007/s40615-016-0326-9

54. Heard-Garris NJ, Cale M, Camaj L, Hamati MC, Dominguez TP. Transmitting trauma: A systematic review of vicarious racism and child health. *Social Science and Medicine 1982*. 2018;199:230–240. doi:10.1016/j.socscimed.2017.04.018

55. Smith BP, Madak-Erdogan Z. Urban neighborhood and residential factors associated with breast cancer in African American women: A systematic review. *Hormones and Cancer*. 2018;9(2):71–81. doi:10.1007/s12672-018-0325-x

56. Castle B, Wendel M, Kerr J, Brooms D, Rollins A. Public health's approach to systemic racism: A systematic literature review. *Journal of Racial & Ethnic Health Disparities*. 2019;6(1):27–36. doi:10.1007/s40615-018-0494-x

57. Forde AT, Crookes DM, Suglia SF, Demmer RT. The weathering hypothesis as an explanation for racial disparities in health: A systematic review. *Annals of Epidemiology.*
2019;33:1–18.e3. doi:10.1016/j.annepidem.2019.02.011

58. Yang TC, Park K, Matthews SA. Racial/ethnic segregation and health disparities:
Future directions and opportunities. *Sociology Compass.* 2020;14(6):e12794. doi:10.1111/
soc4.12794

59. Alson JG, Robinson WR, Pittman L, Doll KM. Incorporating measures of structural racism
into population studies of reproductive health in the United States: A narrative review.
Health Equity. 2021;5(1):49–58. doi:10.1089/heq.2020.0081

60. Rudes G, Fantuzzi C. The association between racism and suicidality among young minority groups: A systematic review. *Journal of Transcultural Nursing.* 2021;33(1):228–238.
doi:10.1177/10436596211046983

2

The Political Determinants of Health and the Race Against Policy-Related Inequities and Determinants (RAPID)

Daniel E. Dawes

Introduction

Entrenched issues related to housing, early childhood and family, and healthcare access, among others, have impacted health equity for generations. Public health and medicine now widely accept a keen understanding that the social determinants of health (SDOH)—where we live, eat, work, play, and pray—all have a tremendous impact on health and wellness. Recognizing that inexorable forces in the environment shape and often determine the health outcomes requires efforts to be focused directly on addressing the fundamental causes and instigators that create those forces, leading to the disparate outcomes seen downstream today. This chapter will examine and illustrate how and why the political determinants of health (PDOH) framework is an innovative and indispensable element of any work that endeavors to truly understand not only the root causes of health inequities, but also the areas within which it will be fruitful to bolster efforts to address these health inequities.

Now, an opportunity exists to ask the pivotal question: to directly address the social and structural conditions that affect health and wellness, are there tangible ways to change the upstream circumstances and factors of which these conditions are mere symptoms? Asserted through a PDOH framework, one can identify, plan, and implement strategies to counter the negative consequences of SDOH that generate the very conditions that give rise to health inequities. Through a PDOH lens, paths can be traced backward from the well-documented disparate health outcomes that occur

Daniel E. Dawes, *The Political Determinants of Health and the Race Against Policy-Related Inequities and Determinants (RAPID)*. In: *Research to Action*. Edited by: Claire Gibbons and Alonzo L. Plough, Oxford University Press. © Robert Wood Johnson Foundation (2026). DOI: 10.1093/9780197819876.003.0003

downstream to their upstream origins, and then ask *what actions, inactions, or decisions created and perpetuated these starting points?* And, just as importantly, ask this of both negative and positive outcomes.

In recent years, public health researchers have increasingly engaged in efforts to move their investigative focuses upstream to discover new interventions that might prevent harm on a large scale. It is imperative to note that PDOH is reflective of this, serving as a step upstream that will *enhance all ongoing efforts moving forward from this date.*

All political determinants affect everyone because they encompass the systematic processes of **structuring relationships, distributing resources**, and **administering power.**[1] However, there are stark differences in how negatively or positively they affect certain individuals and communities. For example, when a transportation policy removes a bus route that runs through a community with residents who heavily rely upon affordable public transportation to get to healthcare appointments, the individuals and families living in that community suffer from a negative political determinant that creates an inequitable resource distribution of public transportation services. Forward-thinking community health centers have launched programs to pay for taxis and/or ride shares to bring people to appointments. However, such efforts—while effective in their immediacy—only treat the symptom, not the root cause of the problem. When such an affected community comes together to advocate for themselves, gathering momentum by convincing more individuals and even local businesses to join their effort, and when they succeed in getting their route reinstated, they have understood the chance to restructure their relationship with the transportation authority. They will have exercised the power inherent in understanding and addressing the political determinants of health.

When the current health inequity challenges are viewed through the PDOH lens, tangible and meaningful steps *within the scope of human control* emerge—actions that can be taken to better, more equitably and justly protect and preserve the health and well-being of everyone. While true, this statement is not meant to suggest that this is an easy or straightforward path. However, the PDOH framework encompasses myriad points of influence within and throughout the social, economic and political systems (e.g., voting, advocacy, commercial interests, government, policy, etc.) that independently and in tandem exert positive or negative pressures on all individuals and communities. In fact, these political determinants very often operate simultaneously in ways that mutually reinforce or influence one another to shape opportunities that either advance health equity or exacerbate health inequities. This ineluctable complexity demands that the political determinants of health be considered in everything that is conceptualized, planned, organized, and implemented to more meaningfully reduce the health and other inequities that plague the nation today. This will require a more in-depth analysis of all research conducted, and of the initiatives and pilot projects funded, because they all need to be undertaken with an awareness of the potential impacts of PDOH.

Context: The Forces Influencing Health, and Getting Out Front with the PDOH Framework[1]

To truly understand these inequities and the impact they are having on population health outcomes, it is important to provide an understanding of the context in which the PDOH exist and permeate throughout society. The effects of political determinants can be observed in many areas of health and healthcare. They include young children growing up without mothers due to high maternal mortality, poor and minoritized families being funneled into substandard housing by inequitable systems, and people across the US struggling to access essential mental healthcare that should be on par with other forms of healthcare. These are only a few abundantly clear examples. At the same time, less obvious upstream factors can begin a domino effect with significant downstream impacts.

The PDOH framework is an important tool because it does much more than explain the origin of health inequities. It can also serve as a guide for making concepts of positive change a reality. Organized into five major areas of focus—**voting**, **government**, **policy**, **advocacy**, and **commercial interests**—the PDOH framework can be used both to identify the drivers of inequity and suggest what can be done in each of the focus areas to create new and concrete opportunities for improvement. Within each of these areas, nuances can be discovered that need to be accounted for in order to employ political determinants proactively in a manner that reduces health inequities, unravels structural racism, and improves the culture of health in the United States. The promise is captivating, but there is much work to be done. While each of the main areas of the PDOH framework is distinct, they are inextricably linked. As such, they should be visualized as a web of influences rather than a single linear process.

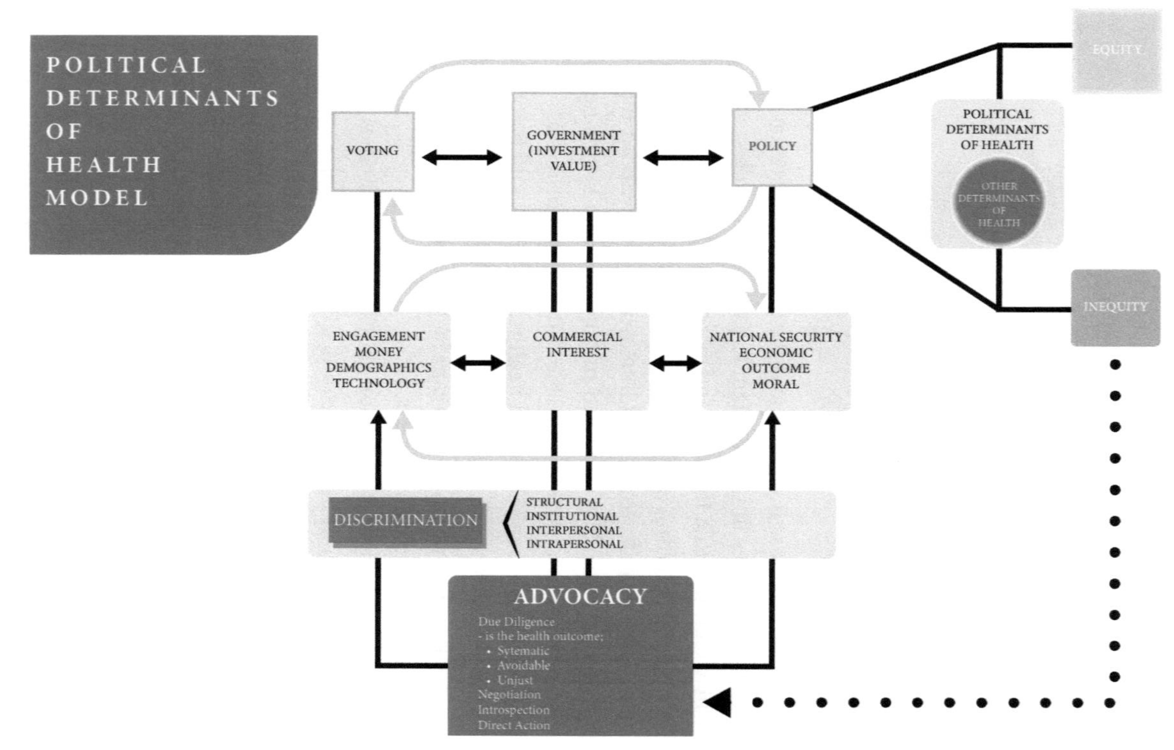

POLITICAL
DETERMINANTS
OF
HEALTH
MODEL
EQUITY
INEQUITY
POLITICAL DETERMINANTS OF HEALTH
OTHER DETERMINANTS OF HEALTH
VOTING
GOVERNMENT (INVESTMENT VALUE)
POLICY
ENGAGEMENT MONEY DEMOGRAPHICS TECHNOLOGY
COMMERCIAL INTEREST
NATIONAL SECURITY ECONOMIC OUTCOME MORAL
DISCRIMINATION
STRUCTURAL INSTITUTIONAL INTERPERSONAL INTRAPERSONAL
ADVOCACY
Due Diligence
- is the health outcome;
• Sytematic
• Avoidable
• Unjust
Negotiation
Introspection
Direct Action

Voting

While many people do not recognize voting's impact on their health, well-being and life expectancy, it may be the most vital of the political determinants. Voting has been consistently associated with better health outcomes, and *not* voting has been consistently associated with poor health. America's numerous political districts and diversity of voting practices do make it difficult to follow a thread from cause to effect. Nonetheless, there are many suggestive correlations. For example, in the *10* least healthy states, voting participation is nearly *10* percentage points lower than in the *10* healthiest states.[2] Fortunately, there are places that offer excellent real-world applications for the direct effect of voting on the health of families and early childhood outcomes.

In a study conducted in Brazil by Thomas Fujiwara and cited by Aliya Bhatia of Vot-ER, when improved voting processes were implemented across the country, it created a natural experiment with astonishingly clear results. The change "promoted a large de facto enfranchisement of mainly less educated citizens." Roughly 10 percent more votes were counted in areas with the new voting processes and in those same places, votes led to 34 percent more funding availability for health programs. As a direct result, prenatal visits increased, which led to a noted decrease in the incidence of low birthweight among Brazil's poorest citizens.[3]

The domino effect that voting begins as a political determinant of health goes well beyond the individual voter. When the Voting Rights Act of 1965 was passed in the United States, for example, the Black–White disparities in the rates of infant mortality narrowed.[3] Further, a recent publication found that the statute led to the enfranchisement of historically marginalized and minoritized populations, bolstering participation in collective decision making, which commonly resulted in reduced inequities experienced by those same groups.[4]

With the powerful connection between voting and health, it's not surprising, then, that research has acknowledged voter suppression as a determinant of racial health disparities.[5] For example, the simple closure of a polling place or adoption of stringent identification requirements to register to vote could have significant negative impacts on the health and well-being of individuals and communities. While this shows the danger of voter disenfranchisement, it also demonstrates the potential that the country holds if more people understood how the political determinants of health profoundly affect lives.[6] Additionally, heightened awareness about how political decisions directly affect the health of individuals and communities sheds light on the fact that increased voter participation can either reinforce or dismantle, and change the root causes of health inequities. In fact, "when Black, Indigenous, Latinx, and Asian American communities are well organized, the act of voting can disrupt the status quo and create a shift to the art of possible, helping to shape the powers that govern their lives."[7]

Policy

The policy landscape is richly textured, with an abundance of attempts to solve pressing problems. Issues often arise because policy tends to benefit one group at the expense of another group. It is an area tumultuous with trade-offs, pulled from all directions by the values and priorities of voters, lobbyists, political strategists, donors, alliances, compromises, and policymakers. At its worst, policy causes tangible harm. However, even well-intentioned policies—even the ones that seemingly work well—can exacerbate inequities. As recently described in the paper *Policy Approaches to Advancing Health Equity*, by Mary Hall (MPH), Corinne Graffunder, (DrPH), and Marilyn Metzler (MPH, RN), "policy interventions can impact communities differently and, in some cases, can widen health disparities. There is some evidence that 'downstream' interventions, which focus on change at the individual level, are more likely to increase health inequality than are 'upstream' interventions, which focus on social change or policy change."[8]

The PDOH framework, therefore, strengthens the analyses of public policies across sectors that have known health implications. Additionally, it centralizes both the direct and indirect policy influences on health and wellness that originate from outside of the traditional healthcare and public health sectors. Studies have confirmed, for example, that educational attainment has a direct impact on the health and wellness of an individual. In fact, in assessing education interventions, the US Community Preventive Services Task Force found that the policy to enact "full-day" kindergarten programs and high school completion alternatives for students at increased risk for non-completion[8] have improved the health prospects of low-income and racial and ethnic minority children and adolescents. Clearly, applying a PDOH lens to educational policies and their impact on health equity is critical to explore today.

Education policies that widen the gap in funding between schools in districts with a high concentration of poor students and those with high concentrations of wealthier students are akin to housing policies that place low-income and minoritized families in substandard housing in unsafe neighborhoods and communities. Clear benefits can be observed in students who had access to expanded free breakfast and lunch during the height of the COVID-19 pandemic, but now those policies are ending. It takes little imagination to guess who will feel the lack of meals most.[9,10]

Throughout every policy realm are powerful examples of the active web of connections that comprise the PDOH framework. For example, policymakers are influenced, in part, by voters, who are influenced, in turn, by their experiences and needs. Add in organizations and their lobbyists, and/or advocacy organizations, and it becomes clear that there isn't a linear flow; there is no single "beginning" of the process in the real world. Instead, there are the constantly fluid processes of push and pull, and give and take to elevate priorities and protect interests.

Advocacy

The power of the people does not sleep between elections. Potent political advocacy can come from grassroots collaborators or elite organizations. Advocacy connects directly to policy and government on one extreme, and to on-the-ground conditions on the other. It might aim to influence policymakers, voters, or even corporations, and it may work subtly, behind the curtain of politics.

More recently, a diversity of stakeholders—dismayed by children being drawn to the fruity flavors and addictive nicotine of Juul's vaping products—took a stand and made the effort to address the policies that were fueling such results. As Nathaniel Weixel reported in *The Hill*, "the FDA has faced growing pressure to regulate vaping as e-cigarette use has skyrocketed among youth and teenagers."[11] The intense and coordinated pressure campaign from parents, educators and public health professionals was a pivotal force that pushed the FDA to remove Juul's products from the US market.[11-13]

One key example of this was the drafting and eventual passage of the land-mark health reform bill, the Affordable Care Act, which included a robust health equity agenda. It was significantly influenced by a consortium of advocates who came together to make sure that health equity and mental health would be prioritized in the final bill. In the end, the bill expanded health coverage to millions of Americans, included 62 health equity-focused provisions, and elevated mental health as a core feature.[11]

When challenges are analyzed using a PDOH framework, it is not only the negative aspects that are magnified; opportunities to achieve signifi-cant positive changes and advancements through advocacy are revealed. For example, when water treatment facilities failed in Jackson, Mississippi in the late summer of 2022, numerous factors of blame were identified. However, one unified response came from Jackson residents, even as K-12 schools and Jackson State University (JSU), an HBCU, had to close in-person educa-tion. It was the parents, students, and educators who banded together and launched a multi-pronged strategy to take direct action to improve their dire circumstances. A middle-school teacher organized a letter-writing cam-paign to the state legislature, urging immediate action to fix water treatment pumps. Simultaneously, JSU students led a water drive to purchase clean drinking water, and university administrators used their position to request comprehensive studies of short- and long-term plans to resolve Jackson's ongoing water problems, and funding to carry out those plans.

Examples such as these point to the need for research, education, and action around advocacy. A stronger understanding is needed of how dif-ferent types of advocacy influence government actions, the downstream effects of those efforts on equitable health outcomes, and the practices at all levels—from those led by leading organizations and individuals to those at the grassroots level—that result in effective use of the political determinants as proactive tools for health equity that sit in the hands of the people.

Commercial Interests

Corporations hold enormous power in the United States, and their inter-ests are frequently protected and advanced in policies and regulations that can have deleterious or beneficial effects on population health. This influ-ence may be seen in the co-location of industrial facilities and low-income housing, environmental safety issues, marketing practices, specific harmful products, pricing of key products, and pushback against or support for regulations by lobbyists. It also can lead to a lack of transparency[12] among experts, or "key opinion leaders," who tend to align with the interests of their key supporters and financial sponsors.[13]

Observed over the last few years are both the dire health and rising economic burdens of chronic disease, which the ongoing COVID-19 pandemic has only exacerbated. With an undue share of the toll being paid by those who were already marginalized before the pandemic, it can be expected to see rising disparities in health outcomes and inequitable financial burdens on the people who are least capable of carrying them.[14]

The national mood tends to brighten when the stock market is on the rise, even though the significant gains tend to be enjoyed primarily by corporations and wealthy individuals. While productivity and economic gains rise, wage growth has lagged behind significantly since the late 1970s, when Milton Friedman introduced the principle of *shareholder primacy*, claiming that the only "social responsibility of business is to increase its profits." Political decisions such as the regulation (or deregulation) of financial institutions have allowed business practices that created a playing field in which not only do traditionally marginalized groups face an uphill battle—most Americans are climbing that same hill. All of this results in an economy that feels precarious for a growing number of middle- and lower-income people and families.[16]

Meanwhile, inflation has proven to be a regressive weight around the necks of America's lower-income population, with the cost of essential items like groceries rising. Unfortunately, its cure may hit even harder. In fact, Jerome Powell, chairman of the Federal Reserve, recently made remarks that are widely viewed as a warning that our bitter pill will come in the form of higher unemployment.[17]

Commercial interests are apparent when companies lobby for preferential treatment or lower corporate taxes, or against transparency laws. When private equity[15] firms own hospitals or physician groups and reduce staffing ratios, purchase the cheapest supplies available, and create burnout among healthcare professionals, those practices can lead to clearly inequitable and disparate health outcomes.[16] However, the view of commercial interests is broad, encompassing the efforts of individual companies and distinct industries to encapsulate the full landscape in which all commercial operations exist.

Taken together, the commercial determinants of health present a multifaceted range of challenges and opportunities. The understanding of PDOH must be leveraged to ensure that commercial interests not only benefit the nation's privileged individuals and communities but also serve the nation's lower-income and minoritized individuals and communities. Dynamics arising from lobbying, business practices, and pressures from corporate boards, investors, employees, trade associations, and others determine whether commercial interests will yield significant advancements in privilege and power to those who already enjoy such benefits or inure to the benefit of all.

When the Volvo car company introduced the three-point seatbelt in 1959, its inventor Nils Bohlin was better known for his work designing ejector seats for fighter planes. Not only did this invention revolutionize safety in Volvo's line of cars, the "company allowed other manufacturers to have the design free of cost, all in the name of safety. At the time of his death in 2002, Volvo estimated that Bohlin's invention had saved more than one million lives in just four decades." This is a shining example of a commercial interest using its power for the benefit of all, and it is easy to see this act as the one that enabled the eventual adoption of laws concerning seatbelts in cars and their use by motorists, where they continue to save thousands of lives each year.[17]

With great power comes great responsibility. This raises the question: how much good could be done by harnessing America's massive engine of commercial activity for the benefit of health equity? History shows that health equity advances have only been possible when they were palatable to commercial interests and had a demonstrable investment value for the government. Considerable work is needed to better understand the many trade-offs and intersecting variables in play in this area. To address it, multi-disciplinary teams must center the essential PDOH questions, even in analyses that do not—on their face—seem related to health and well-being and thus do not appear to pose health-related questions to investigate. See Appendix 1 for the full list of essential PDOH questions.

Government

If a government exists to serve its citizens, it has an unrivaled potential and enduring responsibility to protect their health and well-being. A direct line can be drawn from government-funded research to new vaccines and medications, for example. Notable is the influence of government agencies when they enforce regulations or prioritize public health and safety. However, that power is wielded in partial darkness if we fail to reflect on the complexity of government's operation as a potent political determinant of health.

In Jackson, Mississippi, ongoing water system challenges—including broken pipes, lax safety and sanitation protocols, and temporary boil orders—are not new to the residents who live and work there. In fact, these problems have been growing since the period of White Flight shifted significant portions of Jackson's wealthier residents to its outlying suburbs in neighboring counties. As the tax base deteriorated, the city could no longer keep up with infrastructure maintenance needs. The city of roughly 164,000 residents—82 percent of whom are Black—requested funds for water and sewer repairs on numerous, documented occasions. Legislators in the state legislature, despite the well-known need, blocked the funding requests. The city then requested funds from the American Rescue Plan for the same purposes, but the state requires municipalities to come up with matching funds for such requests, further limiting poor cities and communities like Jackson. Finally, after Jackson's water treatment pumps failed, sending some residents to the hospital with bacterial infections from showering in and inadvertently consuming the putrid water, the Governor declared an emergency, triggering the federal government to get involved and provide immediate help to Jackson. Every step in this process represents a nuance in the way government works, and particularly how it works in Mississippi. It includes skewed dynamics between the local, state, and federal governments, with rules that deleteriously limit the ability of Jackson's governments to satisfy its responsibility to protect its residents.

In Jackson, we see the full complexity of political determinants on display. Residents took action through multiple PDOH nodes, most notably advocacy, voting, and local government, but many of those efforts fell

continued

continued

---

short of their aim for reasons that show the negative potential of political determinants clearly. When the esteemed scholar David K. Jones analyzed political determinants in Mississippi, he found "Systemic barriers to power, including structural racism, [suggesting] that policies that would advance health equity cannot happen without the support of white residents, particularly those living in other parts of the state. In other words, health equity is not likely to be achieved without buy-in from leaders outside the area with the greatest need."

When looking at these complicated situations, the PDOH framework can help to paint a comprehensive picture of cause and effect. In a study conducted by Montez and colleagues, the examination of state policy contexts and the effects of political polarization on population health revealed the well-known divergence in life expectancy between states, which resulted from many factors. As recently as the 1970s, life expectancy was headed closer to parity among states. But in the 1980s, things began to change. In 1960, life expectancies in Oklahoma and Connecticut were exactly the same: 71 years. However, in the span of 60 years since then, Connecticut has improved to 81 years (as of 2018), while Oklahoma rose to just 76 years. From an equal starting point, one state rose to fifth place among the 50 states, while the other fell to 46th.

The authors found that policy bundling—a practice in which different states begin to follow increasingly uniform sets of policies that align with their national partisan identity—created environments and scenarios in which either progressive or conservative ideas have a strong hold. For example, one state might raise the minimum wage to keep up with inflation, enhance the tobacco tax, and allow localities to create paid sick leave policies, aligning with progressive political ideas. However, another state might decline to raise the minimum wage, introduce right-to-work laws, and refuse to expand Medicaid, lining up behind a conservative political identity. In these contexts, one can more easily understand why life expectancy might grow in one state considerably more than another, despite similar starting points.

The Judicial branch can provide a necessary check on potentially harmful rules and statutes. However, recent decisions, such as the failure to secure equitable voting rights for all citizens will result in backslides in Americans' health, with the majority of the losses being felt by Black and other minoritized people. Studies have shown that any restriction of voting rights, such as strict ID laws, reduction of polling places, and restrictions on Sunday voting disproportionately reduce turnout among Black and Latino voters. The clear link demonstrated between increases in voter turnout among poor and minoritized communities and health gains indicates the commensurate losses that will be suffered when votes are suppressed if such regulations are allowed by the highest courts.[17] Even more direct in impact is the overturning of *Roe v Wade*, and its expected tragic threats to the health of women, infants, and families in states that take advantage of that decision by further restricting abortion access. Imagine if the judiciary—both federally and within the states—understood its role among the political determinants of health and questioned rules like those in Mississippi that held back the local government in Jackson from accessing the support they needed for so long.

Under normal circumstances, it is difficult for a city like Jackson to access the resources needed to shore up aging infrastructure. Even in an emergency, there remains a danger that help will be unfairly distributed. A former FEMA administrator describes the practice of distributing emergency funds to places that lost the most value, rather than to the places that need the help the most. In this way, structural racism that causes disinvestment in Black and brown neighborhoods and cities sets those areas up for failure under an ostensibly "color blind" rubric that prioritizes assistance based on the monetary value of affected infrastructure. Craig Fugate, a FEMA administrator under Obama, noted, "Whether it's Appalachia or what we're seeing in Jackson, Mississippi, or in Flint, Michigan, our infrastructure investments have not kept up with the changing risks. Our investments need to be looked at through the lens of where are the most vulnerable populations, not necessarily where are the most valuable properties."[18] The interaction between local, state, and federal governments and their respective priorities, strategies, tactics, rules, and practices to determine the impact on real people living with real needs needs to be better understood. Only then can actionable lessons for advocacy, policy development, commercial interests, governance, and voter education be identified.

It is incumbent upon those of us committed to improving the lives and health of *all* Americans to continue to work, even in places and around issues that may be uncomfortable and are short of allies. The PDOH framework provides non-partisan analytical tools that can and should be used to help find common ground and common goals, and set the nation on a stronger path that leads to health equity. Connecting across party affiliations can be difficult. However, on issues like Medicaid expansion, the benefits are felt by everyone who gains health coverage and by their circles of family and loved ones. The larger healthcare system and all of its players also feel the benefits because Medicaid expansion improves the economic health of states. These benefits are felt regardless of political identity.

The governance contexts in which Americans live affect access to healthcare, housing, quality schools, a living wage, and opportunities for advancement. These distinct, but interdependent determinants of health sit in the very core of how the government works. The PDOH framework, therefore, can be employed to ask the necessary questions about the inner workings of governments. Investigating these questions will give us the opportunity to determine if there are practices, policies, priorities, strategies, tactics, or rules that act as cornerstones in building more beneficial and equitable outcomes, or that stand in the way of those ends.

Implications: Leading by Example

It is easy to make the mistake of thinking that the problems that result in inequities throughout society, and especially to inequity in health, can be solved simply by identifying the drivers and broadcasting this discovery far and wide. However, communication scholars have clarified that information deficit is rarely the true problem. In actuality, solutions are much more difficult to negotiate because there are variances in legitimate political perspectives. Along that broad continuum of perspectives, *not everyone is on the same page and that's okay.* For example, when one person values health above all other priorities and another values fiscal conservatism or crime reduction above all others, finding a balance and common ground can be extremely difficult. There are people who understand the word "equity" to be a code word or concept that means an effort is designed to take resources away from people who earned them to give them to others who seemingly have not. However, there is hope in identifying shared values or goals, and those can be identified and addressed through the PDOH framework. The PDOH model offers a lens to help explore a causal link between a political determinant and an outcome.

For a useful example, we can revisit state governments that have declined to expand Medicaid and then curtailed legal abortions since *Roe v Wade* was overturned. With reduced access to necessary care, maternal mortality is expected to rise. Additionally, we know that when maternal mortality rises, infant mortality rates unfortunately tend to follow. Even when people disagree about government spending on healthcare, we may find prioritizing the health and lives of infants to be common ground that helps us move forward. Another useful example is captured in the land-mark study by Dawes and colleagues, *The Economic Burden of Mental Health Inequities in the United States.*[20] It describes the economic burden associated with inequitable mental healthcare in an argument that will appeal to both fiscal conservatives and equity-minded progressives.

Using the PDOH lens can also help policymakers, voters, business lead-ers, and regulators better understand how every action is a choice that may enhance or inhibit health equity. At the very least, it should be understood that there is a duty to make such choices knowingly. Studies will be needed to show concrete connections between choices and their health outcomes, both positive and negative. For example, what were the health impacts of reducing bus routes, increasing police presence in a particular neighborhood, adding or removing a polling place, making fruit-flavored vape products widely available and accessible, funding municipal water infrastructure, and decid-ing whether or not to vote in an election? These are a mere few examples that apply to and affect all people, to an extent that can be investigated further through a PDOH framework.

A Roadmap to Health Equity: How Communities and Institutions Can Leverage the Political Determinants of Health to Create Systemic Change

To do something profound and meaningful in the advancement of health equity, one must begin by acknowledging and centralizing the political determinants of health in its plans, programs, and organizational culture. Federal agencies, community-serving organizations, and local governments have begun to adopt the PDOH framework for both their respective analyses and proactive work toward health equity. However, to truly understand the web of interconnected determinants, it is necessary that communities, with a comprehensive vision of what is possible, step forward as both innovative leaders and as examples for others to follow.

Call to Action 1: Integrating the PDOH Framework and Essential Questions to Strengthen and Advance all Projects

Recognizing the central importance of the political determinants in virtually all health inequities, the most important call to action is for organizations to commit to include the political determinants in and throughout their respective scopes of work. This can take the form of a project specifically designed to address one or more political determinants, a deep-dive study into a single area of the PDOH model, or ensuring that, at minimum, a project that explores inequities in health outcomes, social, or economic conditions asks, investigates, and analyzes the essential PDOH questions, which are discussed further in Appendix 1.

Call to Action 2: Prioritizing and Demanding Data Equity as a Best Practice for Research—Unraveling PDOH's Wide Web

Researchers exploring health inequities have and will continue to generate considerable volumes of data. However, data collection, reporting, and standardization must be conducted with an understanding of data equity. This is critical because it will ensure that all groups are represented in and by the data gathered, that as much diversity as possible exists on research teams, and that practices (e.g., allowing self-identification consistently) can help capture subtleties that would otherwise be missed, causing data to be misleading and/or less reliable. Other issues to focus on include indigenous data sovereignty and knowledge of the ways in which bureaucracy can and has created barriers to equitable data collection practices. Best practices in data equity should be established to guide all research.

Call to Action 3: Functional Data Platform

PDOH-related inquiries and data generated, or the relevant portions thereof, must be captured, managed, and made easily accessible in a centralized system. Such a robust data system would allow for more inputs, and analyses from many angles, while also ensuring that relevant data and information are available to be more thoroughly investigated in a wide range of future inquiries and research relative to PDOH. If these data can be further democratized by being made available, free of charge, to all researchers, it could spur significant leaps forward in health equity research.

Call to Action 4: Data Analysis: Extracting Value

A multi-disciplinary team should be built to conduct and facilitate ongoing analyses that can generate deeper, more nuanced understandings of the mechanisms by which the political determinants benefit or harm society. Additionally, this dynamic team should leverage the value of asking and addressing the essential PDOH questions across a breadth of research projects to reveal undeniable evidence that can be used to justify policies, practices, and other approaches to dismantling structural racism and improving health equity.

Call to Action 5: Catalyzing Comprehensive Collaboratives

Comprehensive collaboratives will be needed to proactively address structural racism that was born through political determinants upstream and the effects on health equity downstream. Some communities have the power to convene national and local agencies, governments, renowned national associations and organizations, and other thought leaders, but it will be essential that these communities act strongly in concert to catalyze these significant collaborative efforts. This will require strategic and purposeful partnership and alliance development, celebration of milestones, and coordination of networks and efforts across every node in the PDOH framework—government, voting, advocacy, commercial interests, and policy. This strategy is already being explored in St. Petersburg, Florida where the local government was inspired to address political determinants of health and began by publicly recognizing systemic racism as a public health crisis.[19,20]

Call to Action 6: Building the PDOH-Enabled Workforce

Each community should build a workforce that is equipped to employ the PDOH framework in its day-to-day work. First, it is important to look across the five core areas of the framework and develop communication and education strategies that can meet potential partners where they are whether they are a scholar, community leader, policymaker, or community member.

One potent opportunity is to use exceptional relationships (for, e.g., schools of public health and academic health institutions) to establish opportunities for diverse, transdisciplinary junior faculty and community leaders to participate in and lead PDOH-centered projects in their areas of expertise. This will simultaneously magnify efforts to address political determinants of health, fill the data repository mentioned above, and nurture the next generation of public health and health equity leaders. There is no shortage of work to be done in this arena.[21]

Call to Action 7: Training: Boots on the Ground

Short, accessible training modules and programs should be developed for individuals in each of the five core areas of the PDOH framework to teach them how to understand their work and the context of their lives to better equip them to take a hands-on role in mitigating negative political determinants and leveraging positive political determinants.

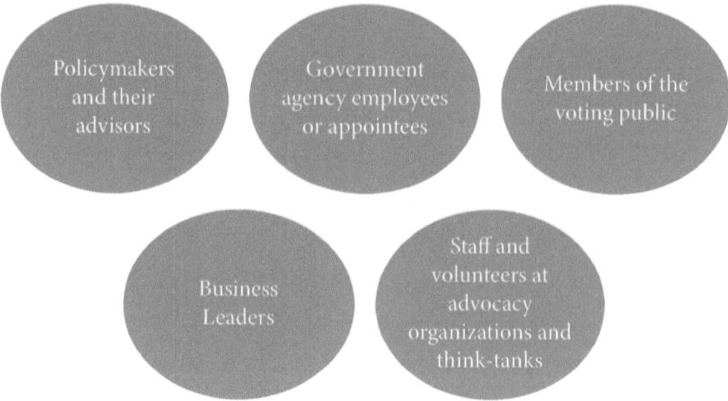

With these training modules and programs, organizations will have an arsenal of effective and applicable tools to build strategic partnerships with allies working in challenging and difficult spaces. These tools will also prepare partners who are already enthusiastic about dismantling structural racism and promoting health equity to address the determinants of the determinants through their existing and future work.

Call to Action 8: Amplify Communications
& Dissemination Strategy

Using every partner and communication channel available, every organization should capitalize on the concrete and applicable PDOH model to encourage broad-based initiatives and actions. Through existing work, it is known that the professional and scholarly community is often only waiting to be asked to help and collaborate. *Put out the call.* Of equal importance is to strategize in order to communicate as effectively outside the bubble of their respective areas as within.

By making an effort to educate public-facing authorities in the media, there is an opportunity to make enormous strides through informing voters and advocacy groups of the principles defined by the PDOH framework. Using strategic science communications principles and convening peer organizations and national influencers will have the effect of increasing public awareness of and knowledge about the positive influence and great potential of the PDOH model. Advertising companies have been helping companies influence the public's view of the world for generations, and it is time to learn something from them. Engaging not only those experts in the academy, but also those with marketing and advertising experience to learn the principles of persuasive and effective communication with the public will be a significant step forward for the organization's efforts to shift the way Americans think about their health and well-being, and that of their communities.

Conclusion: Connecting the Dots

The political determinants of health reveal the concrete underpinnings of problems well-known and revealed via the social determinants of health. For a generation, it has been known that the context in which humans live, eat, work, play, and pray has an outsized impact on health. It is also known that those determinants drive innumerable health inequities, but little attention has been paid to the instigators of the social determinants of health or the *fundamental causes of the causes.* The PDOH framework is more than just another way to view problems around inequities; it is a tool with which anybody who sees health inequity can understand how to operate within their own role to create positive change. With a PDOH framework, humanity can now begin to be more proactive and effective. It creates a scenario where the pursuit of solutions continually fights the current to travel further and further upstream until thoughtful and sound answers to complicated questions are generated.

The organizations and communities defining the health equity landscape over the next decades should employ the PDOH framework to recognize and influence these powerful drivers if they want to realize actionable results.

Doing so will allow historically and currently marginalized and vulnerable communities around the country to benefit from the bipartite goal of dismantling structural racism and achieving true health equity.

Appendix 1: The Essential PDOH Questions

In all venues, especially those not explicitly focused on PDOH, there is an opportunity to consider how political determinants may function or interact with the effects being studied, interventions being implemented, business practices, and so on. The essential PDOH questions are a simple set of questions that provide a methodical approach for those who wish to ensure their work addresses the positive and negative potential represented by the model.

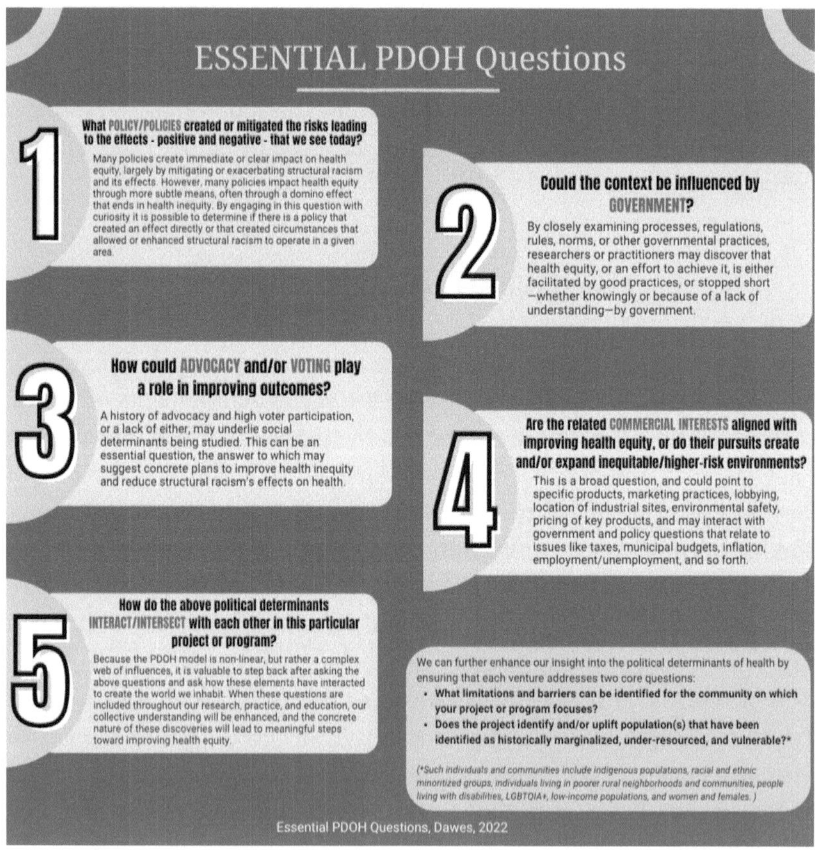

References

1. Dawes DE. *The political determinants of health*. Baltimore, MD: Johns Hopkins University Press; 2020.
2. Ehlinger EP, Nevarez CR. Safe and accessible voting: The role of public health. *American Journal of Public Health*. 2021;111(1):45–46. doi:10.2105/AJPH.2020.306011
3. Fujiwara T. Voting technology, political responsiveness, and infant health: Evidence from Brazil. *Econometrica*. 2015;83(2):423–464. doi:10.3982/ECTA11520
4. Hahn RA, Truman BI, Williams DR. Civil rights as determinants of public health and racial and ethnic health equity: Health care, education, employment, and housing in the United States. *SSM—Population Health*. 2018;4:17–24. doi:10.1016/j.ssmph.2017.10.006
5. HIng AK. The right to vote, the right to health: Voter suppression as a determinant of racial health disparities. *Journal of Health Disparities Research and Practice*. 2018;12(6). https://digitalscholarship.unlv.edu/jhdrp/vol12/iss6/5/.
6. Yagoda N. Addressing health disparities through voter engagement. *Annals of Family Medicine*. 2019;17(5):459–461. doi:10.1370/afm.2441
7. Robert Wood Johnson Foundation, Vaidya A, Poo A, National Domestic Workers Alliance, Brown L, Black Voters Matter. Why community power is fundamental to advancing racial and health equity. *NAM Perspectives*. 2022;6. doi:10.31478/202206b
8. Hall M, Graffunder C, Metzler M. Policy approaches to advancing health equity. *Journal of Public Health Management Practice*. 2016. doi: 10.1097/PHH.0000000000000365
9. Campoamor D. Universal free lunch has ended: "Students can't learn if they're hungry." *Today*. September 1, 2022. https://www.today.com/parents/parents/universal-free-lunch-ends-rcna43827?querylydemo=related.
10. Masenthin T. Free meals for all students will end in August; Lawrence school board to set meal prices. *The Lawrence Times*. June 29, 2022. https://lawrencekstimes.com/2022/06/29/student-meal-prices-lawrence/.
11. Dawes DE. *150 years of Obamacare*. Baltimore, MD: Johns Hopkins University Press; 2016.
12. Heneghan C, McCartney M. Declaring interests and restoring trust in medicine. *British Medical Journal*. November 6, 2019:l6236. doi:10.1136/bmj.l6236
13. Moynihan R, Macdonald H, Heneghan C, Bero L, Godlee F. Commercial interests, transparency, and independence: A call for submissions. *British Medical Journal*. April 16, 2019:l1706. doi:10.1136/bmj.l1706
14. Singhal S, Patel N. The future of US healthcare: What's next for the industry post-COVID-19. McKinsey & Company. July 19, 2022. https://www.mckinsey.com/industries/health care-systems-and-services/our-insights/the-future-of-us-healthcare-whats-next-for-the-industry-post-covid-19.
15. Farmer B. Buy a rural hospital for $100? Investors pick up struggling institutions for pennies. *NPR*. August 16, 2022. https://www.npr.org/sections/health-shots/2022/08/16/1116960419/buy-a-rural-hospital-for-100-investors-pick-up-struggling-institutions-for-penni.
16. Olson LK. *Ethically challenged: Private equity storms US health care*. Baltimore, MD: Johns Hopkins University Press; 2022.
17. Brennan Center For Justice. The impact of voter suppression on communities of color. January 10, 2022. https://www.brennancenter.org/our-work/research-reports/impact-voter-suppression-communities-color.
18. Hennessy-Fiske M. White then Black residents abandoned Jackson, propelling its water crisis. *The Washington Post*. September 4, 2022. https://www.washingtonpost.com/nation/2022/09/04/jackson-water-crisis/.

19. American Public Health Association (APHA). *Structural Racism is a Public Health Crisis: Impact on the Black Community*; 2020. https://www.apha.org/policy-and-advocacy/public-health-policy-briefs/policy-database/2021/01/13/structural-racism-is-a-public-health-crisis

20. American Public Health Association (APHA). *Racism Declarations.* Accessed November 17, 2025. https://www.apha.org/topics-and-issues/racial-equity/racism-declarations

21. Dawes D, Amador CM, Jha M, et al. *The economic burden of mental health inequities in the United States report.* Satcher Health Leadership Institute at Morehouse School of Medicine; 2022. https://satcherinstitute.org/wp-content/uploads/2022/09/The-Economic-Burden-of-Mental-Health-Inequities-in-the-US-Report-Final-single-pages.V6.pdf.

3

Health, Wealth, and Structural Interconnected Drivers of Racial Health Disparities

William Darity Jr., Keisha L. Bentley-Edwards, Lauren Brinkley-Rubinstein, Raffi E. García, Nicholas Datto, Morgan Maner, Salama S. Freed, Arjumand Siddiqi, and Tiffany Green

The growth in interest and attention to the social determinants of health disparities has led to socioeconomic status (SES) being assigned a central role in explaining racially unequal health outcomes. Socioeconomic status typically has been defined based on an individual's or household's income, educational attainment, or occupational position. Customarily, less notice has been given to another key potential facet of SES, wealth.

Furthermore, structural racism is a fundamental process generating racially disparate health outcomes. In turn, the Black–White disparity in wealth is the integral element of structural racism, producing disproportionate pressures on Black families, leading to comparatively depressed levels of physical and mental well-being.

Racial inequality in wealth is more than a "mediating factor" between structural racism and disparate health outcomes. It is the touchstone indicator of the degree of structural racism, operating as a root cause of other disparities in well-being, including health outcomes. Darity, Mullen, and Slaughter have described "the Black–White wealth gap . . . as the single-most appropriate measure of the cumulative intergenerational impact of White racism on [living] descendants of" persons enslaved in the United States (p. 117).[1]

The objective of this chapter is to illuminate what, currently, is known about the relationships between health, wealth, and structural racism, to indicate what more needs to be learned, and to offer recommendations for policy, research, and health systems.

William Darity Jr. et al., *Health, Wealth, and Structural Interconnected Drivers of Racial Health Disparities*. In: *Research to Action*. Edited by: Claire Gibbons and Alonzo L. Plough, Oxford University Press. © Robert Wood Johnson Foundation (2026). DOI: 10.1093/9780197819876.003.0004

Structural Racism, Wealth, and Health Disparities

An existing and established literature has sought to understand persistent racial inequities in health in America. Racial disparities are particularly prominent with respect to longevity,[2] heart disease,[3] and cancer.[4] While there have been gains overall in life expectancy and infant mortality among Whites and Blacks, the White–Black relative gap remains stable and substantial.[4]

In addition, Black people face higher levels of health-damaging stress, have less access to healthcare, experience lower rates of utilization of healthcare,[5] and are beset by discrimination while seeking and receiving care.[6] Recently, scholars have focused on structural racism as a cause of these disparities in health, with a particular focus on conditions of residential segregation, gaps in income, and educational inequality.[4,7]

Structural racism has been defined as "the totality of ways in which societies foster [racial] discrimination, via mutually reinforcing [inequitable] systems . . . (e.g., in housing, education, employment, earnings, benefits, credit, media, healthcare, criminal justice) that in turn reinforce discriminatory beliefs, values, and distribution of resources," reflected in history, culture, and interconnected institutions.[8,9] Structural racism is embedded in systems to create advantages for a dominant racial group at the direct or indirect expense of marginalized "others."

These inequitable systems that "reinforce discriminatory beliefs, values, and distribution of resources" are manifest in public policies related to housing, employment, and distribution of wealth. Thus, structural racism casts systemic conditions as the root source of racial inequality, in opposition to the perspective that treats racial inequality as a consequence of group-based differences in cultural practices and behavior.

Structural racism affects people at the levels of both the population and the individual, and the extant literature has identified systems that embody the harms: the criminal legal system (disproportionate police contact, jail and prison incarceration, and probation and parole), housing and residential segregation, and healthcare and medical institutions.[9,10] Underlying these conditions are the processes that influence the acquisition and maintenance of wealth, particularly the intergenerational transmission of resources.[11]

The Particular Role of Wealth

Structural racism has a clear and lasting impact on health. Its presence and impact are captured powerfully by an individual's ability to accumulate wealth. This intersection of structural racism, wealth, and health is particularly important to disentangle, as we attempt to more clearly identify how wealth interacts with health to produce and intensify persistent racial health inequities.

Income and wealth are distinct concepts. Income is a flow of resources received on a regular basis, generally from earnings, interest generated by owned assets, sale of an asset, or transferred payments. Wealth is a stock of resources, assets minus debts (or liabilities), *net worth*, or the net value of an individual's, household's, or organization's property. An asset is a resource owned by an individual, household, or organization, a potential source of future income to meet debts, facilitate additional accumulation of property, or meet other commitments. A debt is money owed or due to another party.

The absolute magnitude of the racial wealth gap depends on whether it is measured at the median or the mean. Estimates from the 2019 Survey of Consumer Finances (pre-pandemic) placed the absolute dollar value of the Black–White difference in median household net worth at a substantial $164,100, while the absolute dollar value in the Black–White difference in mean (or "average") net worth was a much larger $840,900.[12]

Students of inequality generally prefer to focus on median values because, in large samples, they are more representative of the typical experience of members of each group under comparison. However, for two reasons, it is more appropriate to focus on mean values when the racial wealth gap is under consideration.

First, because the wealth distribution is so heavily skewed toward the top, *97 percent of the wealth held by White households is owned by those with a net worth above the White median.*[13] As a result, the conventional emphasis on the median gap deflects attention from a vast amount of the wealth held by White households. Second, the concentration of wealth among White households above the White median is not due solely to the wealth possessed by a handful of extraordinarily rich White billionaires. One-quarter of all White households have a net worth exceeding $1 million, while that is true for only

4 percent of Black households.[13] Indeed, while members of the White professional managerial class have a median net worth about three times as high as members of the White working class (e.g., $276,000 versus $114,270 in 2019), members of the White working class have a median net worth two to three times as high as members of the Black professional managerial class (e.g., $114,270 versus $38,800 in 2019). Of course, Black working-class wealth is significantly lower than all others.[14]

These racial disparities in wealth originated with an array of policies conducted by the US government that built White wealth while blocking Black wealth accumulation. After slavery, the federal government failed to meet the promise made to the Freedmen of 40-acre land grants as restitution for the years of bondage. Simultaneously, under the auspices of the Homestead Act of 1862, 160-acre land grants were given to 1.5 million White families, resulting in benefits for at least 45 million living White Americans.[15]

Compounding the wealth disparity effects of the racial asymmetry in land allocation, the federal government was complicit in or ignored upward of 100 White massacres directed at Black communities from the end of the Civil War to World War II that led to the loss of Black lives and the appropriation and seizure of Black property. In the twentieth century, Congress shifted from asset-building via land distribution to asset-building via homeownership promotion, but homeownership supports were discriminatorily applied, including the redlining policies pursued by the Federal Housing Administration in conjunction with private banks across the country and the uneven application of the business and homeownership provisions of the G.I. Bill.

In the latter half of the twentieth century, federal funds for freeway construction were used to build highways that, selectively, were located down the center of Black communities, destroying Black business districts.[16,17] Federal policies forged the racial wealth gap in the United States, a disparity magnified across generations.

Because the racial differential in net worth, the wealth disparity, is primarily a product of transmission of resources across generations—and hence "inherited"—it is a fundamental characteristic of structural racism, rather than merely a mediating factor. See Figure 3.1. Even the racial *income* gap for the current adult generation is, significantly, a partial product of the disparate *wealth* position of Black and White parents and grandparents, respectively.[18]

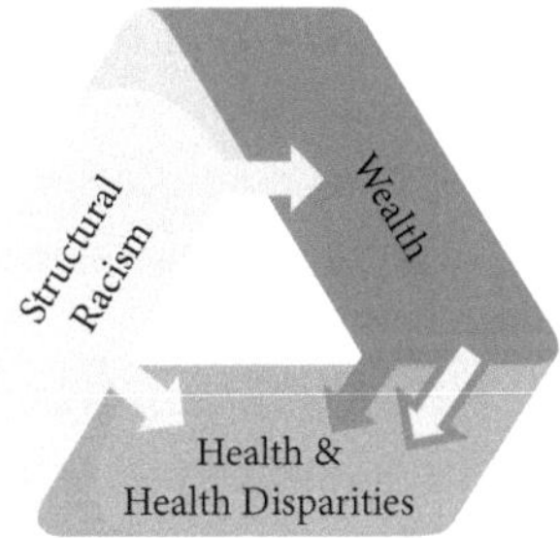

Figure 3.1 The direct and indirect influence of structural racism and wealth on health

Race, Wealth, and Health

The relationship between health and wealth is complex. Lum[19] found that there was a significant, unidirectional association between and from health to wealth moderated by race and ethnicity. The association between health and change in net worth was positive and nonmonotonic for older White people. For older Black people, this association was negative and nonmonotonic.

A limitation of this study, and several others we discuss below, is that it examines the relationship between current wealth and current health within a generation without accounting for the inherent simultaneity. Fully treating racial wealth differences as a fundamental dimension of structural racism necessitates looking at the relationship between the previous generation's wealth and the younger generation's health.

Individuals with less than a high school education report higher household debt in excess of assets and higher incidence of hypertension, coronary heart disease, and diabetes than individuals with higher education levels.[20]

Differences in the prevalence of chronic conditions between racial groups and their potential attribution to differences in socioeconomic status are also apparent. Black individuals are less likely to own their place of residence than White respondents, and they have significantly lower housing and nonhousing wealth. These differences in SES largely map onto differences in health status for racial groups.[21]

An analysis of PSID data[22] connects institutional racism to disparities among Black individuals' health and wealth statuses. Health is measured by six self-reported outcomes: self-rated health, chronic conditions, work limitations, disability risk, psychological distress, and body mass index. Wealth was measured as household net worth (total assets minus total debts) in 2015; to identify the association between other components of wealth and health outcomes, home equity, cash savings, stocks, and debt were analyzed as well.

Black participants had worse health than Whites across self-rated health, nearly seven times that of Black participants; greater home equity, savings, and financial assets; and were nearly twice as likely to own a home.[22] White participants carried more debt, but, arguably, more often, the type of debt that could generate asset building in the future.

Women face unique barriers to obtaining and accessing wealth. Recurring financial strain is associated with a decline in health during middle and later life, especially for those women who reported recurrent strain. Favorable changes in household income and household wealth do not eliminate these effects due to accumulated financial strain.[23]

A bidirectional relationship between health and wealth—assessed in this study as the sum of debts for each household minus total household assets, age (independent of marital status and employment), and partner's health[24]—characterizes the impact of wealth on older Black women's health and found that there was not a statistically significant association between self-rated health and wealth despite a difference of approximately $75,000 between individuals reporting the very best and very worst health outcomes. However, findings indicated that there was a significant correlation with earnings and education, particularly for individuals with higher levels of education.[25]

Racial-ethnic disparities in cardiovascular conditions and risk factors do not mirror SES disparities (including wealth, measured here as a participant's homeownership and assets) in the same conditions, and Black–White disparities in cardiovascular conditions and risk factors vary considerably by gender. Cardiovascular conditions bear a complex relationship with education-based social inequities.

Individuals with lower education levels report higher household debts in excess of income and wealth, and a higher incidence of hypertension, coronary heart disease, diabetes, and psychiatric problems than participants with higher education levels.[20] Individuals with higher education levels are likely to have more access to healthcare, and thus, the total effects of excess debt are likely an underestimate of the true education-based inequalities in health outcomes.

One study explored the effect of dementia on wealth disparity in Black versus non-Black Americans using HRS data.[26] Dementia was found to be associated with a loss of 97 percent of wealth among Black Americans, compared with 42 percent among non-Black Americans. Wealth loss among Black and non-Black Americans without dementia was not statistically different.[26] This study is important because of its focus on factors specific to older adults, who have had a lifetime to accumulate wealth. Regardless, whether wealth is measured at the median or the mean, the racial gap widens markedly with age.[27]

Recommendations for Policy, Research, and Health Systems

Structural racism has specific influences on both health and wealth, as can be seen through the differing relationships between the two variables based on the intersection of race, gender, and age. In the American context, structural racism is implanted in law, policies, and the enforcement of these policies from its founding to contemporary contexts.[28,29] The persistent and evolving nature of structural racism, and the resulting outcome disparities, can feel insurmountable.

We argue that eliminating disparities in health and wealth, while also developing ubiquitous positive outcomes, can only happen with equally persistent and evolving measures that fight structural racism. The following research recommendations provide strategies for best practices in assessing and centering race, gender, and class in understanding the relationship between wealth and health. The government and health system policy recommendations offer bold initiatives that address and remediate the role of structural racism on both wealth and health outcomes.

Research Recommendations

Using Race in Research

This chapter emphasizes the importance of using racial variables in analysis. However, we also argue that race and ethnicity variables must be used in ways that accurately and ethically respond to research questions. Although health is a biological concern, race should be understood as a social construct. Race is not based on genetics, nor purely based on physical attributes, but is defined by the members of the community *and* the power structures that enforce racial distinctions.[30,31]

The social construction of race supports the racial hierarchies that are indicative of structural racism. Thus, the disparities we see along racial lines represent the exchange between social constructs that influence outcomes in health and wealth, rather than genetic causes. It is important to understand if your analytical model is evaluating different racial experiences that lead to specific outcomes (appropriate) or if you are using (biological) race as the cause for outcomes (inappropriate).

Ultimately, researchers should be clear about what is meant when examining the role of race on outcomes, particularly since race and many sociodemographic status indicators are closely related (e.g., Whiteness and high wealth status). To be clear, while race is a social construct, it still has very real influences on outcomes. **Researchers may avoid including race or treating race as a focus of research to avoid the appearance of making claims of inherent racial differences;[32,33] however, the absence of relevant racial variables diminishes the scholarly rigor of relevant research.**

When making comparisons across race, the comparison group should be clearly identified and explained. There is a long history of using White people as the reference group due both to systems of social power and due to the tendency of viewing White experiences as normal, neutral, or the standard. At times, this may be appropriate when evaluating disparities between the dominant racial group in America with marginalized "others."

Yet, depending on the question of interest, analytical strategy, and diversity of the participant pool, it may be more prudent to make the mean/median of the overall population level statistic the referent to better demonstrate both disadvantages *and* advantages in outcomes. *So, it is not just a matter of African Americans facing a greater burden of heart disease-related morbidity and mortality than White people, it is also recognizing that White Americans face a health advantage in heart disease-related morbidity and mortality.* This approach makes clear when structural racism may be at play and requires deeper inquiry. Research, and specifically statistics, is neither race-neutral nor color-blind. Additionally, as more people identify with a multiracial identity, it is imperative that researchers do not force participants to choose only one race *and* analyze the participants based on how they identify.

Comparing Apples to Apples: The Importance of Disaggregated Data

How can you understand the intersection of race on health and wealth outcomes if research doesn't compare similarly situated people? If we know that White Americans have substantially more median and mean wealth than their counterparts of other racial and ethnic groups, merely comparing differences in health does not offer sufficient explanations. This becomes apparent when seeking linear relationships between wealth and health across racial groups.

For example, when Hajat and colleagues[34] used the Panel Study of Income Dynamics (PSID), they found that eight times more White than non-White people were in the highest wealth quintile, while there were 10 percent more non-White than White people in the poorest wealth category. Their findings of relative risk of cardiovascular disease factors for those in the highest wealth quintile are skewed by the predominant racial makeup of this group (White).

So, while it is clear that low and high wealth have indications for financial and environmental resources that inform health outcomes, it is not clear how these indicators may function differently by race. We recommend that studies collect or utilize robust data on standard demographic variables, gender, race/ethnicity, earnings, income, marital status, educational attainment, work experience, training, and family size with strong representations at the intersections through oversampling.

Strong disaggregated data also provides opportunities for robust within-race research. Within-race research, or those that only include data from a specific racial/ethnic group, acknowledges the diversity of experiences and backgrounds for these groups. Further, we also recommend within-race research because it helps to determine what factors provide the greatest benefit or harm for that group—which is vital information to have when developing interventions and policies.

Measuring Structural Racism

We have proposed throughout this chapter that structural racism can be measured effectively by the Black–White wealth gap. The racial wealth differential provides a spare but powerful indicator of the extent to which a society fosters inequality. This contrasts sharply with the strategy advanced by Hardeman and colleagues[35] in which a legion of measures is advanced to operationalize the concept of structural racism. The all-in approach introduces a set of measures of structural racism that potentially conflate cause and effect, for example, residential segregation, employment discrimination, and even health disparities themselves. Essentially, the measurements often focus on the consequences rather than the source of structural racism. These measures are also potentially highly intercorrelated. If they are used via construction of an index, there is a significant loss of information about the relationship with any individual component of index, but if each measure is included separately in an analysis, it will reduce the degrees of freedom, adversely affecting the strength of tests for statistical significance.

Ultimately, while our inclination is to lean toward the racial wealth gap as the best measure of structural racism, we recognize there is a need for additional research that establishes which measure or combination of measures is most effective in explaining disparities in health outcomes.

Measuring Health

How we ask participants about their health has practical implications for research and how we interpret the findings. There are benefits and drawbacks to utilizing self-rated/subjective health or clinical/objective measures, depending on the resources available to researchers. Self-rated health is an important measure of health and a strong predictor of mortality,[36–38] but it is challenged by age and cultural connotations of health, as well as health literacy concerns.

When using self-rated health assessments, researchers need to clearly define what is meant by "health." For example, is health seen as the ability to perform everyday functions, work, or engage in recreational but strenuous activities like riding a bike or running?

Conversely, objective (e.g., have you been diagnosed with … ?) or clinical data (gathered from a practitioner or medical records) can be costly, time-consuming, or difficult to acquire due to institutional review board (IRB) and privacy constraints. We recommend that whenever possible, researchers utilize a blend of self-rated and objective/clinical measures of health.

A recurring concern in the health/wealth research is that most of the existing national datasets either have rich data on wealth *or* health. Although the

PSID has the best representation of both wealth and health,[38] the racial distribution in the wealth distribution is a concern. A national data set with strong racial representation across the wealth spectrum that includes subjective and objective health measures is needed to gain a better understanding of the health-wealth connections across racial groups.

Government-based Health Policy Recommendations

Policies that address racial health equity while also considering wealth must be intentional in their approach. In the past, both research and policy focused on (low) income and other socioeconomic factors as a proxy for race in their initiatives. Some use this approach for political expediency because they do not feel they will receive support from fellow legislators or the public, or for the perception of color-blind solutions.[39] Others believe that social class is more predictive than race on health outcomes—often to avoid discussions of racism. We argue that the issue at hand is structural racism. As such, **structural racism infiltrates the experiences and outcomes of individuals to create benefits and cause harms across social class strata.** There are structural barriers to obtaining healthcare services that are indirectly tied to structural racism. For example, property values and the wealth gap due to redlining policies factor into the availability of healthcare providers. Even as healthcare delivery systems continue to innovate and find new ways to deliver care, the advances are not evenly distributed and often benefit the wealthiest individuals over others.

Access to Healthcare

A clear example of this exists with Urgent Care Clinics and Retail Clinics. Often billed as an alternative to care in the physician's office or emergency department, these clinics provide similar services, but on a walk-in basis and for lower costs than emergency department services. While it seems these clinics would expand access to healthcare services, the location of clinics actually reduces access to services; these clinics are disproportionately located in wealthy areas. This means Urgent Care and Retail Clinics increase access for wealthy individuals who already have access to care, while those who are not wealthy and are not conveniently located near an Urgent Care or Retail Clinic still do not have access to the care they need. The lack of care access is especially detrimental in rural areas. Additionally, large cities and rural communities alike have been impacted by Medicare-enforced desegregation in the 1960s and the contemporary refusal to expand Medicaid, resulting in hospitals shutting down in places with high medical needs.[40,41] Beyond the lack of healthcare facilities, there is a shortage of primary care and specialty providers in general, and specifically Black providers. This shortage also extends to vision, dental, hearing, and mental health services. There are a few ways in which we can remedy this disparity. First, we must find a way to incentivize healthcare systems to locate and remain in healthcare deserts. The federal government must address the loss of rural and urban hospitals and providers due to this change in policy.

Second, parity between payment rates between Medicaid, Medicare, and private insurance would contribute greatly to the increasing provider density in healthcare deserts. Programs exist that incentivize primary care providers to practice in rural areas in exchange for student loan forgiveness. However, upon receipt of this loan forgiveness and completion of the program, many of the providers move to areas with higher patient volume and payment rates. Finally, expanding beyond just physician care by increasing the scope of practice for nurse practitioners and dental therapists in rural areas would greatly reduce disparities in access to care.

Universal Health Coverage

Policies and initiatives must be intentional and steadfast to counter the enduring effects of structural racism on health. Quick solutions may improve individual lives—and of course, individual lives are important. However, moving the needle on population-level health disparities requires bold, population-level approaches. Similarly, initiatives that seek to address racial disparities must center racial dynamics and racism specifically to be effective.

Health insurance that is untethered to work or income status has gained popularity and holds promise to improve overall population-level health outcomes. However, universal health policies may not eliminate health disparities on their own. With universal approaches, a rising tide lifts all boats. As seen with the overall improvements in infant and maternal care, mortality rates for these groups have also improved overall. Yet the Black–White racial disparities in infant and maternal deaths have remained two to one for decades.[42,43] This is in part because access to care is one very big contributor to racial health disparities, but quality of care is also a significant source of concern.

Howell and colleagues[44] estimated that were Black women in New York City to deliver in the same hospitals (an access issue) *and* receive the same quality of care, very low-birth weight infant survival would improve, and the Black–White infant mortality disparity would decrease by 34 percent. We recommend that the adoption of universal programs must also include a provision of equal access to high specialty healthcare facilities and monitoring to ensure that patients are receiving care based on effective practice standards.

Eliminating the Racial Wealth Gap

To the extent that wealth disparities affect health disparities, a potential route toward reducing Black–White differences in health outcomes can be the elimination of the racial wealth gap. Three major approaches have been advanced to accomplish the goal: universal programs that will disproportionately increase Black American net worth, Black-specific programs that indirectly lower the differential in Black and White wealth, and Black-specific programs that directly lower the differential in Black and White wealth.

We will argue here that the first two strategies are likely to be least effective in erasing the gulf in wealth between Blacks and Whites, while the third strategy, appropriately designed, can be fully effective in closing the racial wealth gap. In the first category—universal programs that, ostensibly, will give a disproportionate boost to Black wealth—we include student debt cancellation, tuition-free education at public institutions of higher education, and baby bonds. In the second category—indirect strategies—are specific support for Black-owned businesses, funds for historically Black colleges and universities, and subsidies to promote Black homeownership. The third and final category is best described as a plan for Black reparations.

To be clear, the efficacy of any proposal intended to lower the racial wealth gap is dependent upon the measure used to determine the magnitude of the gap. The estimated effectiveness of any proposal for erasing the racial wealth gap is sensitive to the targeted amount. The two major options for targets are the Black–White difference in median wealth and the Black–White difference in mean wealth; in 2019 based upon the Survey of Consumer Finances, the former amounted to $164,000 and the latter amounted to $840,900 per household.

Accounting for differences in average household size—2.37 persons per White household and 2.47 persons per Black household—the per-person racial gap came to about $68,000 at the median and $350,000 at the mean. As a result, we argue that the more appropriate target is the larger one, measured at the mean.

Student Debt Cancellation

Under the first category, student debt cancellation has been touted as a mechanism for achieving a significant reduction in the racial wealth disparity.[45] It is clear that Blacks who have enrolled in college or university have a higher average level of student loan debt than White enrollees, $23,400 versus $16,000, although the average level of total indebtedness held by Blacks is significantly less than average White total wealth.[46,1] Adjusting for the higher White college enrollment rate, and given the fact that both Blacks and Whites would incur a wealth gain from student loan erasure, the net reduction in the wealth gap will amount to $1864, a mere three percent of the difference at the median and an infinitesimal drop at the mean.[46]

Indeed, eliminating student loan debt could usher in a zero-tuition world for higher education. Given the universality of the zero-tuition condition, coupled with higher initial White enrollment rates, there would be little direct effect on the racial wealth gap. However, any indirect effect associated with a potential narrowing of racial gaps in educational attainment is likely to be marginal at best. At present, Black heads of household with a college degree have two-thirds of the net worth of White heads of household who never finished high school.[47] Blacks in the professional-managerial class are generally better educated but not only have lower average levels of income but also significantly lower levels of wealth than members of the White working class.[14]

---

[1] A Prosperity Now study in 2019 reported that median total black household liabilities were $30,800, while median White household liabilities were more than twice as large at $73,800. However, White households had a median level of assets valued in excess of $260,000 in contrast with the median Black household's assets valued at $55,900. The median Black household had 40 percent of the debt of the median White household, but only 20 percent of the assets. Correspondingly, the ratio of assets to debts for Black households was 1.6 versus 2.8 for white households, both measured at the median.

Baby Bonds

"Baby bonds" also have been proposed as a universal program that, ostensibly, will close the racial wealth gap. Not actually a "bond," the plan would give each newborn infant a government funded trust account, calibrated based on their parents' wealth position, that they could access when they reached the legal age of maturity, or a bit later in young adulthood.

Because Black children typically are born into families with low or negative wealth, their average increase in wealth will be greater than the increase for White children. Baby bonds have been designed to bring every American child's wealth position close to the national median level of net worth, and this feature of the plan especially limits its effectiveness when the goal is to eliminate the racial wealth gap at the mean.

To give the efficacy of baby bonds full rein, we consider their impact in a world 35–40 years beyond its inception; since young people can only access the funds 18–20 years after their birth, the full effects of the program will not be felt until a generation later. The estimated average benefit per White child will be an increase in net worth of about $33,000 and about $55,000 per Black child, a net reduction in the gap of $22,000.[48]

While hardly closing the racial wealth gap in entirety, a fully executed baby bonds plan would lower the differential at the median by a substantial nearly 30 percent. In contrast, at the mean, it would lower the differential by less than 10 percent. Baby bonds, tuition-free college, and student debt relief are all good ideas. But their proponents need to be more circumspect about what they can accomplish in addressing the Black–White difference in wealth.

Support for Black-owned Businesses the Racial Wealth Gap

Next, we consider policies that are put forward as indirectly closing the racial wealth gap. The most prominent of these are monetary supports for Black businesses. The premise here is that Black business development will have spread effects, increasing wealth across the Black community.

Mehrsa Baradaran's study of the history of Black banking and the concept of Black capitalism indicates that there is no assurance that uplift for Black enterprise will lead to community-wide uplift among Black people.[49] Moreover, a persuasive argument can be made that in order for Black businesses to develop more fully, baseline wealth in the Black community must be raised, enabling more Black entrepreneurs to shoulder more risk, to sustain their businesses during difficult times, and to expand and grow existing businesses; that is, you increase Black wealth to raise Black business development, rather than vice versa.

What is evident is that the task of building Black enterprise to a scale that approximates the scope of White-owned enterprise is a staggering mission, perhaps one of mythical proportions. The 21 Black-owned banks have less than $5 billion in total assets; JPMorgan Chase alone has in excess of $3 trillion in assets. All Black-owned businesses combined have less than half of the annual retail sales of Walmart alone. Only 4 percent of Black-owned businesses have more than one employee, including the owner.[10] Prior to 2020, there were approximately 2.6 million Black-owned businesses—this number significantly declined with the onset of the COVID-19 pandemic. Still, if a program of Black business subsidies doubled Black retail sales, the total still would trail Walmart.

Funds for Historically Black Colleges and Universities

Funds for historically Black colleges and universities (HBCUs) should take the form of building their relatively small endowments. It would not take extravagant sums of money to significantly improve their endowment positions. The 10 HBCUs with the largest endowments have a total of approximately $2 billion, while a single historically White institution like Smith College has a similar-sized endowment. An outlay of $100 billion to HBCUs could have a meaningful impact on the stability and success of Black colleges and universities.[50]

Presumably, financially stronger institutions will enroll more Black students, thus enhancing the educational profile for younger Black Americans. But what are the implications for the racial wealth gap? Since the link between reducing educational disparities and reducing net worth disparities is tenuous, it is unlikely there will be much of an effect. Intergenerational transmission of resources far dominates educational attainment as a factor determining an individual's, a family's, or a household's level of wealth.

Another point to consider is that Black students comprise roughly 75 percent of students at most HBCUs, with some having a higher or lower percentage of non-Black students (e.g., 90 percent of Bluefield State College's students are White). Programs that benefit HBCUs will not solely benefit Black students. Stronger HBCUs are a desirable goal, but the consequences for Black–White wealth inequality are mild at best.

Increasing Home Ownership

The goal of housing subsidies for Black Americans is to bridge the racial disparity in homeownership. Rates of homeownership now stand at roughly 74 percent for Whites and 45 percent for Blacks. If we were to eliminate the disparity in a climate where there is a huge, discriminatory differential in the equity value of homes, amounting to $50–100,000, the component of the wealth gap associated with homeownership would remain large.[50]

Under plans proposed put forward during the 2019 phase of the Presidential election, using a combination of homeownership rate equalization and equity equalization, a set of generous assumptions led to an estimate of a $67,800 gain in net worth for Black American households.[50] If there was no effect on the White homeownership position, this would constitute a fairly robust 40 percent drop in the Black–White wealth gap at the median, but it would amount to less than a 10 percent drop in the Black–White wealth gap at the mean.

There also is an unfortunate tendency to overemphasize, even romanticize, the significance of homeownership as *the* key asset in an American portfolio. This overemphasis downplays the importance of non-residential property, business ownership, stocks, bonds, and other financial assets, and retirement accounts. Closing the wealth gap with respect to homeownership alone takes 65–75 percent of the average portfolio out of consideration.

What happens if we combine all of these policies and implement them to full effect simultaneously? On the most optimistic count, at the median, 70–75 percent of the racial wealth gap can be eliminated. Proponents could declare victory or, at least, near victory. However, if the target is set more appropriately at the mean, 70–75 percent of the racial wealth gap will remain untouched.

Reparations

The final set of proposals—directly attacking the racial wealth gap by providing payments to Black Americans sufficient to erase the differential—also has different implications if the goal is to bridge the median or the mean difference in net worth. If there are about 40 million Black Americans whose ancestors were enslaved in the United States who would be eligible for payments, the amount required would be about $3 trillion, a large sum but well within the range of the expenditures the federal government made in response to the pandemic, via the CARES Act and the American Rescue Plan.

The median gap is the more conservative target, and it is the target that omits 97 percent of the wealth held by White Americans out of consideration.

Bridging the racial wealth gap at the mean would require an expenditure closer to $14 trillion, which, if it were spent all at once by its recipients, could trigger massive inflation. There are two ways in which a bill of that magnitude can be met. First, the payments could be spread out across multiple years, preferably no longer than a decade. Second, the payment need not be made exclusively as cash transfers. They could take the form of less liquid assets, including trust accounts and annuities. The key principle here is that eligible recipients should have full discretion over the use of the funds, just as other recipients of restitution from the American government have had in the past, for example, Japanese Americans who received redress payments for unjust mass incarceration during World War II.[28]

Indeed, what is being described here is a program of reparations for Black American descendants of US slavery, given the significance of the wealth gap as the prime economic indicator of the cumulative, intergenerational effects of American racism. *Would reparations have beneficial effects on health outcomes?* One recent study suggests that in the absence of a Black–White wealth gap, transmission rates of COVID-19 would have been 31 to 68 percent lower.[51] Two recent commentaries in medical/health sciences journals call for greater attention to be given to the potential health benefits of reparations, understood as closing the racial wealth gap.[52,53]. When considering specific health impacts, the type of asset used to meet the reparations bill matters. Attentiveness to the health effects of closing the racial wealth gap can have implications for the asset composition of the payments made to eligible recipients. But it is apparent that closing the racial wealth gap alone will not fully close the racial health gap. In what follows, we explore additional policies that can further the cause of reducing Black–White disparities in health.

Health System Recommendations

Often, discussions of structural racism focus on government-level policies, while ignoring that structural racism also works between and within interlocking systems and workplaces.[54] Health systems are not excluded from the execution and maintenance of structural racism. Health systems include organizations of providers and trainees, administrators, hospitals, and care facilities with shared policies and practices for the delivery of healthcare.

Research co-sponsored by the Robert Wood Johnson Foundation[55] revealed how care experiences were informed by healthcare experiences. Their findings revealed that 22 percent of the Black, 17 percent of the Latinx, 9 percent of Asian American and 15 percent of the Native American adults in their study avoided going to the doctor for fear of discrimination, as opposed to 3 percent of White adults. What makes this information distinctive is that when disaggregated, much of the White participants' mistrust of the healthcare system was based on sexual orientation/gender identity or for being low income. None of the high-income White adults feared discrimination in healthcare settings. African American and Latinx participants' fear of discrimination did not waiver based on income status. These findings point to the need to address racism in healthcare settings directly.

Healthcare mistrust is not only about interpersonal discrimination or mistreatment. That institutions allow these individual-level racist encounters to occur without repercussions is indicative of structural racism. Individual racism can only survive if it is supported by the systems in which it operates. Therefore, policies can't stop at implicit bias training to solve these issues.[56,57]

Moving Beyond Implicit Bias

Health systems must examine their policies and practices that support racially disparate outcomes and serve as contributors to structural racism. A commitment to a meaningful racial landscape analysis requires sufficient funding for staff, programs, and evaluations, as well as ardent support from senior leadership. By monitoring their morbidity and mortality records, referrals, and complaints, health systems can identify areas where bias exists in the system, including in their care algorithms and especially their race correction practices.

A highly effective way to reduce the gap in health outcomes would be to eliminate the bias due to race correction that permeates the US healthcare system. This race correction is baked into kidney, pulmonary, and osteoporosis screenings, to name a few.[58] Race correction, or race norming, is the longstanding and increasingly unpopular practice of adjusting clinical guidelines for patients based upon race or ethnicity. These guidelines determine the point at which medical intervention is necessary and usually require a greater threshold for Black people. The race correction factors are not based on inherent genetic differences between races. In fact, the correction factors are borne of faulty and racist assumptions about marginalized populations.[58-60]

A recent study of the impact of the race correction factor on chronic kidney disease (CKD) diagnoses found that if the results of Black patients' kidney function screenings had been judged without the race corrector, more than one-third of the authors' study population would have been reclassified to a more severe stage of chronic kidney disease. This discrepancy has widespread consequences: Black people are less likely to receive the treatment necessary to prevent the advancement to End-Stage Renal Disease (ESRD) and are also less likely to be referred for a transplant in a timely manner.[61,62]

Racial disparities in ESRD and CKD staging are but one example of the negative effects of utilizing the race correction factor; the downstream consequences of race correction are persistent throughout the healthcare system. Elimination of these factors, or at the very least revisiting the scientific justification for using these factors, would have a substantial impact on achieving racial parity in healthcare.[58] Although race correction is being re-evaluated, and in some cases, rescinded as a part of standards of care by several medical associations, it is unclear how much race-correction practices remain within health systems.[63]

After monitoring their policies and practices, and biases are revealed, health systems must engage in evidence-based remedies and interventions from the interpersonal to system levels to address these biases. New and existing racism remediation strategies require continuous tracking and adjustments. Meaningful, rather than incremental progress should be prioritized. Before eliminating thoughtfully formulated interventions, health systems should evaluate whether amendments can be made. Eliminating a structural racism remediation strategy prematurely due to opposition or slow return on investment can be counterproductive or demoralizing. As such, health system leaders who are dedicated to eliminating structural racism must be intentional in their actions and stand firm in their values.[64] As such, leaders should be prepared for resistance to changing the status quo that may be familiar yet is directly or passively causing racial health disparities.

Conclusion

When considering the influence of wealth on health outcomes, race matters—more specifically, racism matters (see Figure 3.1). In this chapter, we revealed how wealth is not a race-neutral indicator of health. Structural racism influences wealth and health outcomes. Still, wealth has crystallized as a specific health determinant with benefits and detriments that functions differently across race. Whether the goal is to eliminate health inequities or the racial wealth gap, structural racism cannot be tackled using passive approaches. Structural racism evolves over generations, often at the same pace as racial progress. It is imperative that remedies to health and wealth inequities are of significant magnitude to affect not only individual outcomes, but also, more importantly, to create systemic and intergenerational solutions.

References

1. Darity Jr W, Mullen AK, Slaughter M. The cumulative costs of racism and the bill for Black reparations. *Journal of Economic Perspectives*. 2022;36(2):99–122.
2. Levine RS, Foster JE, Fullilove RE, et al. Black–white inequalities in mortality and life expectancy, 1933–1999: Implications for healthy people 2010. *Public Health Reports*. 2001;116(5):474.
3. Vaughan AS, Quick H, Pathak EB, Kramer MR, Casper M. Disparities in temporal and geographic patterns of declining heart disease mortality by race and sex in the United States, 1973–2010. *Journal of the American Heart Association*. 2015;4(12):e002567.
4. Williams DR, Jackson PB. Social sources of racial disparities in health. *Health Affairs*. 2005;24(2):325–334.
5. Berchick ER, Hood E, Barnett JC. *Health insurance coverage in the United States: 2018*. Washington, DC: US Department of Commerce; 2019.
6. Maina IW, Belton TD, Ginzberg S, Singh A, Johnson TJ. A decade of studying implicit racial/ethnic bias in healthcare providers using the implicit association test. *Social Science & Medicine*. 2018;199:219–229.
7. Yearby R. Racial disparities in health status and access to healthcare: The continuation of inequality in the United States due to structural racism. *American Journal of Economics and Sociology*. 2018;77(3–4):1113–1152.
8. Bailey ZD, Krieger N, Agénor M, Graves J, Linos N, Bassett MT. Structural racism and health inequities in the USA: Evidence and interventions. *The Lancet*. 2017;389(10077):1453–1463.
9. Bailey ZD, Feldman JM, Bassett MT. How structural racism works: Racist policies as a root cause of US racial health inequities. *Massachusetts Medical Society*; 2021;384(8):768–773. doi:10.1056/NEJMms2025396
10. Darity Jr W, Hamilton D, Paul M, et al. What we get wrong about closing the racial wealth gap. *Samuel DuBois Cook Center on Social Equity and Insight Center for Community Economic Development*. 2018;1(1):1–67.

11. Diette TM, Goldsmith AH, Hamilton D, Darity W. Race, unemployment, and mental health in the USA: What can we infer about the psychological cost of the great recession across racial groups? *Journal of Economics, Race, and Policy*. 2018;1(2):75–91.

12. Bhutta N, Chang AC, Dettling LJ, Hsu JW. Disparities in wealth by race and ethnicity in the 2019 Survey of Consumer Finances. *FEDS Notes*. 2020. https://www.federalreserve.gov/econres/notes/feds-notes/disparities-in-wealth-by-race-and-ethnicity-in-the-2019-survey-of-consumer-finances-20200928.html.

13. Darity Jr W, Addo FR, Smith IZ. A subaltern middle class: The case of the missing "Black bourgeoisie" in America. *Contemporary Economic Policy*. 2021;39(3):494–502.

14. Addo FR, Darity Jr WA. Disparate recoveries: wealth, race, and the working class after the Great Recession. *The ANNALS of the American Academy of Political and Social Science*. 2021;695(1):173–192.

15. Shanks TR. The Homestead Act: A major asset-building policy in American history. In: Sherraden, M., ed. *Inclusion in the American dream: Assets, poverty, and public policy*. Oxford: Oxford University Press; 2005:20–41.

16. Bentley-Edwards KL, Edwards MC, Spence CN, Darity WA, Hamilton D, Perez J. How does it feel to be a problem? The missing Kerner Commission Report. *RSF: The Russell Sage Foundation Journal of the Social Sciences*. 2018;4(6):20–40. doi:10.7758/RSF.2018.4.6.02

17. Darity WA, Mullen AK. Race in America: Reparations. *The Economist*. May 18, 2021.

18. Toney J, Robertson CL. Intergenerational economic mobility and the racial wealth gap. *AEA Papers and Proceedings*. 2021;111:206–210.

19. Lum T. Health-wealth association among older Americans: Racial and ethnic differences. *Social Work Research*. 2004;28(2):105–116. doi:10.1093/swr/28.2.105

20. Batomen B, Sweet E, Nandi A. Social inequalities, debt, and health in the United States. *SSM–Population Health*. 2021;13:100736.

21. Schoenbaum M, Waidmann T. Race, socioeconomic status, and health: Accounting for race differences in health. *Journals of Gerontology Series B*. 1997;52:61–73.

22. Boen C, Keister L, Aronson B. Beyond net worth: Racial differences in wealth portfolios and black–white health inequality across the life course. *Journal of Health and Social Behavior*. 2020;61(2):153–169.

23. Shippee TP, Wilkinson LR, Ferraro KF. Accumulated financial strain and women's health over three decades. *Journals of Gerontology Series B: Psychological Sciences and Social Sciences*. 2012;67(5):585–594.

24. de Brey C, Musu L, McFarland J, et al. *Status and trends in the education of racial and ethnic groups 2018*. Washington, DC: National Center for Education Statistics; 2019.

25. Sharma A. Wealth and the health of older Black women in the United States. *Health Promotion International*. 2019;34(5):1055–1068.

26. Kaufman JE, Gallo WT, Fahs MC. The contribution of dementia to the disparity in family wealth between black and non-black Americans. *Ageing & Society*. 2020;40(2):306–327.

27. Landsberg MH-. How much do racial wealth gaps affect the next generation. 2016. May 3. https://thesocietypages.org/socimages/2016/05/03/how-much-do-racial-wealth-gaps-hurt-the-next-generation/.

28. Darity WA, Mullen AK. *From here to equality: Reparations for black Americans in the twenty-first century*. Chapel Hill: The University of North Carolina Press; 2020.

29. Hannah-Jones N. *The 1619 Project: A new origin story*. New York: Random House Publishing Group; 2021.

30. Yudell M, Roberts D, Desalle R, Tishkoff S. Taking race out of human genetics. *Science*. 2016;351(6273):564–565.

31. Bentley-Edwards KL, Scott M, Robbins PA. How systemic racism and preexisting conditions contributed to COVID-19 disparities for Black Americans. In: Wright G, Darity Jr WA, Hubbard L, eds. *The pandemic divide: How COVID increased inequality in America*. Durham, NC: Duke University Press; 2022:29–45.

32. Roberts SO, Bareket-Shavit C, Dollins FA, Goldie PD, Mortenson E. Racial inequality in psychological research: Trends of the past and recommendations for the future. *Perspectives on Psychological Science.* 2020;15(6):1295–1309.
33. Bonilla-Silva E. The invisible weight of whiteness: The racial grammar of everyday life in contemporary America. Article. *Ethnic & Racial Studies.* 2012;35(2):173–194.
34. Hajat A, Kaufman JS, Rose KM, Siddiqi A, Thomas JC. Do the wealthy have a health advantage? Cardiovascular disease risk factors and wealth. *Social Science & Medicine.* 2010;71(11):1935–1942.
35. Hardeman RR, Homan PA, Chantarat T, Davis BA, Brown TH. Improving the measurement of structural racism to achieve antiracist health policy. *Health Affairs.* 2022;41(2):179–186.
36. Wuorela M, Lavonius S, Salminen M, Vahlberg T, Viitanen M, Viikari L. Self-rated health and objective health status as predictors of all-cause mortality among older people: A prospective study with a 5-, 10-, and 27-year follow-up. *BMC Geriatrics.* 2020;20(1):120. doi:10.1186/s12877-020-01516-9
37. Lorem G, Cook S, Leon DA, Emaus N, Schirmer H. Self-reported health as a predictor of mortality: A cohort study of its relation to other health measurements and observation time. *Scientific Reports.* 2020;10(1):4866. doi:10.1038/s41598-020-61603-0
38. Hajat A, Kaufman JS, Rose KM, Siddiqi A, Thomas JC. Long-term effects of wealth on mortality and self-rated health status. *American Journal of Epidemiology.* 2010;173(2): 192–200.
39. Edwards M, Darity Jr WA. Why color-blind solutions won't solve the racial wealth gap: How we can overcome the Constitutional hurdles to race conscious remedies in addressing the wealth gap. *Kentucky Law Journal.* 2021;110:769.
40. Bentley-Edwards KL. The African American health burden: Disproportionate and unresolved. In: Darity Jr WA, Mullen AK, Hubbard L, eds. *Black reparations: The case for redress and the path to get there.* Oakland, CA: University of California Press; 2023:95–108.
41. Smith DB. *The power to heal: Civil rights, Medicare, and the struggle to transform America's system.* Nashville: Vanderbilt University Press; 2016.
42. Smith IZ, Bentley-Edwards KL, El-Amin S, Darity Jr W. Fighting at birth: Eradicating the Black–White infant mortality gap. 2018:14. https://socialequity.duke.edu/wp-content/ uploads/2019/12/Eradicating-Black-Infant-Mortality-March-2018.pdf.
43. Ramraj C, Siddiqi A, El-Amin S, Hamilton D. What matters more, maternal characteristics or differential returns for having them? Using decomposition analysis to explain Black–White racial disparities in infant mortality in the United States. *Race and Social Problems.* 2019;11(14):282–289. doi:10.1007/s12552-019-09268-x
44. Howell EA, Hebert P, Chatterjee S, Kleinman LC, Chassin MR. Black/white differences in very low birth weight neonatal mortality rates among New York City hospitals. *Pediatrics.* 2008;121(3):e407–e415.
45. Pressley, A. Pressley, Omar, Waters, Adams introduce bold resolution calling on President-Elect Biden to cancel $50,000 in federal student loan debt. December 17, 2021. https://pressley.house.gov/2020/12/17/pressley-omar-waters-adams-introduce-bold-resolution-calling-president-elect/.
46. Darity W. The true cost of closing the country's racial wealth gap. *The New York Times.* April 30, 2021. https://www.nytimes.com/2021/04/30/business/racial-wealth-gap.html.
47. Natasha Hicks FA, Anne Price and William Darity Jr. *Still running up the down escalator: How narratives shape our understanding of racial wealth inequality.* Samuel Dubois Cook Center on Social Equity; 2021. https://socialequity.duke.edu/wp-content/uploads/2021/ 09/INSIGHT_Still-Running-Up-Down-Escalators_vF.pdf.
48. Cassidy C, Heydemann R, Price A, Unah N, Darity Jr W. Baby bonds: A universal path to ensure the next generation has the capital to thrive. 2019. https://socialequity.duke.edu/ wp-content/uploads/2019/12/ICCED-Duke_BabyBonds_December2019-Linked.pdf.

49. Baradaran M. *The color of money: Black banks and the racial wealth gap*. Cambridge, MA: Harvard University Press; 2017.

50. Darity Jr W, Equity S. Running the numbers on closing the racial wealth gap. *Report of the Samuel DuBois Cook Center on Social Equity*, Durham, NC: Duke University; 2019.

51. Richardson ET, Malik MM, Darity Jr WA, et al. Reparations for Black American descendants of persons enslaved in the US and their potential impact on SARS-CoV-2 transmission. *Social Science & Medicine*. 2021;276:113741.

52. Bassett MT, Galea S. Reparations as a public health priority: A strategy for ending black–white health disparities. *New England Journal of Medicine*. 2020;383(22):2101–2103.

53. Wrigley-Field E. US racial inequality may be as deadly as COVID-19. *Proceedings of the National Academy of Sciences*. 2020;117(36):21854–21856.

54. Ray V. A theory of racialized organizations. *American Sociological Review*. 2019;84(1): 26–53.

55. National Public Radio, Robert Wood Johnson Foundation, Harvard T. H. Chan School of Public Health. Discrimination in America: Experiences and views of African Americans. 2017:56. https://www.rwjf.org/en/insights/our-research/2017/10/discrimination-in-america--experiences-and-views.html.

56. Green TL, Zapata JY, Brown HW, Hagiwara N. Rethinking bias to achieve maternal health equity: Changing organizations, not just individuals. *Obstetrics & Gynecology*. May 1 2021;137(5):935–940.

57. Green TL, Hagiwara N. The problem with implicit bias training. *Scientific American*. 2020;31(6): 22.

58. Vyas DA, Eisenstein LG, Jones DS. Hidden in plain sight: Reconsidering the use of race correction in clinical algorithms. *New England Journal of Medicine*. 2020;383(9):874–882.

59. Braun L. Race correction and spirometry. *Chest*. 2021;159(4):1670–1675.

60. Bavli I, Jones DS. Race correction and the x-ray machine: The controversy over increased radiation doses for Black Americans in 1968. *New England Journal of Medicine*. 2022;387(10):947–952.

61. Norris KC, Eneanya ND, Boulware LE. Removal of race from estimates of kidney function: First, do no harm. *Journal of the American Medical Association*. 2021;325(2):135–137.

62. Ahmed S, Nutt CT, Eneanya ND, et al. Examining the potential impact of race multiplier utilization in estimated glomerular filtration rate calculation on African-American care outcomes. *Journal of General Internal Medicine*. 2021;36(2):464–471.

63. National Kidney Foundation, American Society of Nephrology. *Removing race from estimates of kidney function*. March 9, 2021. https://www.kidney.org/press-room/removing-race-estimates-kidney-function.

64. Bentley-Edwards KL, Fleming P, Doherty IA, Whicker D, Mervin-Blake S, Barrett N. The 5Ws of racial equity in research: A framework for applying a racial equity lens throughout the research process. *Health Equity*. 2022;6(1):917–921. doi:10.1089/heq.2022.0042

SECTION II

DOING THE WORK: MEASURING STRUCTURAL RACISM AND APPLYING AN ANTIRACIST LENS

Section II, building knowledge: Innovative approaches to research challenges longstanding assumptions about how scholarly work should be conducted, opening the door to overlooked voices and broader ways of knowing. Recalibrating approaches to evidence gathering does not mean that researchers forego well-established scientific norms but rather that they recognize the limits of traditional approaches and the imperative of forging more inclusive tools. The three chapters in this part look at the art and science of measurement and acknowledge both the opportunities and challenges of generating change-promoting knowledge.

Chapter 4, Measuring Structural Racism: What Do We Know and Where Do We Go? looks at how the intricate ties between structural racism and health equity have been analyzed and why additional robust approaches are needed. A literature review finds that most racialized research focuses on Black populations, often omits older adults, uses residential segregation as a core indicator, and frequently employs neighborhood as the measure of analysis. A cross-sector "barnraising" workshop adds to the knowledge base with ideas about measuring thriving, safeguarding against health equity tourism, and defining and engaging community. The findings yield a package of suggestions for innovative study design and a set of questions to guide funders in advancing the field.

Chapter 5, Lessons from the Urban Institute's Demonstration Projects describes the multi-level, multi-systems structural analysis required to conduct policy-oriented social science research on the relationship between structural racism and health outcomes. Five RWJF-funded demonstration studies conducted by Urban Institute research teams examined policy issues related to transportation, behavioral health, child welfare, taxation, and retirement, and uncovered racial dimensions to all of them. While the research yielded important insights, it also underscored the complexity of questioning assumptions, building trust with partners, and fostering institutional change. Confronting embedded hierarchies, investigating root causes, and taking a cross-disciplinary approach all require nuanced attention.

Chapter 6, Promoting Equity in the Justice System builds on the evidence that vast racial inequities are reflected in every aspect of policing and criminal justice. A literature review and informant interviews also reveal knowledge gaps and suggest that the available data are fragmented, inconsistent, and inadequately disaggregated. Qualitative input gathered from those with lived **experience** will help fill those gaps. Emphasizing diversionary alternatives and public safety over policing, strengthening community supports and health systems, decriminalizing low-level offenses, and confronting implicit biases in justice policy and practice are among the evaluable pathways to shaping a more equitable system.

4

Measuring Structural Racism

What Do We Know and Where Do We Go?

Center for Antiracism Research for Health Equity (CARHE)
at the University of Minnesota

Introduction

Across most health indicators, racial inequities exist in which those from racialized groups have worse health than their White counterparts (racialized communities encompass people who are socially assigned as non-White in race). Medical advances, increased access to healthcare, behavioral interventions, and improvements to nutrition have all been applied to reduce the racial health gap, yet inequities persist despite these efforts. This entrenched reality is a public health crisis, but the tools we use to intervene in this problem too often focus on downstream interventions. Instead, we need to move upstream, addressing the structural factors that shape how risk and resources are distributed across society. Structural factors are those that shape the rules of our society. They are both practices and ideologies that influence how society is organized.[1] A critical upstream factor contributing to racial health inequities is structural racism.

While many definitions of structural racism exist, we prefer the one provided by Bailey and colleagues (2017), who define structural racism as "the totality of ways in which societies foster racial discrimination, through mutually reinforcing inequitable systems (in housing, education, employment, earnings, benefits, credit, media, health care, criminal justice, and so on) that in turn reinforce discriminatory beliefs, values, and distribution of resources, which together affect the risk of adverse health outcomes."[2] The ideology of a racial hierarchy that undergirds the aforementioned "discriminatory beliefs, values, and distribution of resources" is fueled by White supremacy.

Rachel Hardeman, *Measuring Structural Racism*. In: *Research to Action*. Edited by: Claire Gibbons and Alonzo L. Plough, Oxford University Press. © Robert Wood Johnson Foundation (2026). DOI: 10.1093/9780197819876.003.0005

White supremacy is "a society-wide system that removes power from non-white people through means both blatant and invisible; from the daily pangs of interpersonal racism to the subterranean harms of implicit bias in our schools and hospitals to the disparate accumulation of wealth that began in slavery and dispossession, continued in redlining and segregation, and echoes still in unequal household wealth and access to capital."[3] As interlocked and mutually reinforcing systems, structural racism and White supremacy create and maintain the cultural values, policies, practices, rules, and behaviors in our society from individual to institutional to structural levels, upholding advantages for White people while producing systemic disadvantages for racialized communities.

Historically, race was seen as a biological rather than social construct, but antiracist research shifts that framing to focus on *racism*, not race, as a fundamental cause of racial health inequities. A growing body of researchers has begun to link structural racism to racial health inequities, while grounding in further theoretical and conceptual support where empirical evidence is lacking.[1,4-8] However, a key challenge of this research lies in how to operationalize and measure structural racism. In 2018, Groos and colleagues conducted a comprehensive literature review and found that only 20 articles on structural racism and health had been published over the course of 30 years.[9] In 2020, the deaths of George Floyd Jr., Ahmaud Arbery, and Breonna Taylor, along with so many other members of the Black community whose lives were stolen too soon—at the hands of police or due to disproportionate and unjust exposure to COVID-19[10]—catalyzed collective action through uprisings across the country and the world.

As our society grapples with a racial reckoning on the historical and contemporary impact of structural racism and White supremacy on Black people and all racialized people, a deluge of research on structural racism and health has flooded the field. Journals have called for scholarship on structural racism. Institutions have issued statements about antiracism, diversity, equity, and inclusion. Both public and private funders have shifted their funding priorities to support scholarly and community-engaged work to dismantle racism. Many researchers have answered these calls, and from 2019 to 2021, a significant uptick in structural racism research occurred. Additionally, community organizations and non-profit groups have begun discussing how to measure structural racism in their communities. Despite this progress, we are far from having the knowledge and tools to understand how structural racism is connected to health or how to accurately measure structural racism quantitatively.

Comprehensive measures of this complex social construct have been elusive and are an active area of research.[11] Too often, even when structural racism is considered, measures rely on individual perceptions of experiences of discrimination rather than capturing a broader, more upstream, conceptualization of structural racism.[9] This individualistic approach provides an incomplete picture of the many ways in which structural racism manifests across people's lives and underestimates the effect of White supremacy on health. Overall, researchers in this field continue to debate whether existing measures embody what we aim to evaluate.[9]

As health equity researchers, our goal is to conduct research that reduces inequity, contributes to understanding and dismantling structural racism, and reimagines a more equitable society while empowering those most impacted by structural racism. But we cannot change what we cannot measure.[9] Reliable, replicable, and theoretically informed measures of structural racism are required to advance our knowledge of structural racism and health.

This chapter is based on a 2022 report for the Robert Wood Johnson Foundation (RWJF) signature program Evidence for Action (E4A) and summarizes our findings. In it, we provide recommendations for future efforts to understand better the complex mechanisms linking structural racism and racial health inequities.

Methods

As part of our work with RWJF, we investigated structural racism measures and attitudes about those measures in two stages. In **Stage 1**, we conducted a scoping review to examine existing literature on measuring structural racism since Groos and colleagues published their seminal article, Measuring Inequity: A Systematic Review of Methods Used to Quantify Structural Racism in 2018.[9] Scoping reviews are a type of quasi-systematic review used for understanding research on emerging topics that are distributed across published peer-reviewed academic and grey literature or located in different academic disciplines.[12] The scoping review for this study focused on gray and academic literature from 2019 to 2021 to avoid duplicating the work already done by Groos and colleagues, which explored academic literature published from 2007–2017.[9] Given that only published academic literature was reviewed by Groos and colleagues through 2017, we sought to augment that work with gray literature databases and search engines. While the full scoping review will be published elsewhere, in this chapter we will highlight the key themes we observed in this review and how they relate to the current and future state of structural racism measurement.

In **Stage 2**, we conducted a "barnraising" workshop in March 2022. A traditional barnraising in the Midwest is a collective gathering in which a community comes together to build a barn in a short amount of time. In the same way, we asked our measurement community to come together to build toward discussing, refining, and developing measures of structural racism. Our "Improving the Measurement of Structural Racism Barnraising" event convened academic researchers, community leaders, policy and law experts, industry representatives, and data users from across the US to hold conversations about creating and utilizing measures of structural racism as a tool for achieving health equity. In total, 43 participated in the workshop in person and 220 participated virtually. During this one-and-a-half-day workshop, participants engaged in dynamic conversations on how to create and utilize structural racism measures to move the field of health equity research forward. While many of the workshop participants reside in the Minneapolis-Saint Paul area, others traveled from across the country to participate. Scholarships were made available for five out-of-town experts to alleviate their expense burdens to ensure equitable access to knowledge on structural racism measurement. The agenda for the Barnraising can be found in Appendix 1.

Synthesis of Findings

Our review identified 35 articles that measured structural racism from 2019–2021, which was more than triple the number of studies that Groos and colleagues (2018) identified over a previous 10-year period. In comparison to Groos and colleagues (2018), we identified a greater diversity of domains being measured, such as political participation, incarceration, and racialized police encounters. Additional dimensions of segregation in our review were measured across residential segregation, occupational segregation, socioeconomic segregation, economic inequity, housing and mortgages, and incarceration. Several other studies also measured multiple domains of structural racism using a combination of education, housing, economic, environmental, judicial, civic, carceral, and healthcare measures. A summary of common measures used across structural racism studies, though not exhaustive, can be found in Appendix 2.

Based on our review, four themes emerged in how structural racism is being operationalized and measured.

Focus on Anti-Black Racism

In the context of the United States, which is where this chapter focuses its attention, structural racism is often studied through an anti-Black perspective that centers the history of slavery, Jim Crow laws, and overall disproportionate harm inflicted upon Black Americans across multiple domains and all stages of the life-course. Given the entrenched anti-Blackness in American society, structural racism is a clear contributing factor to enduring health inequities for Black Americans, making it a primary subject of investigation for health researchers and practitioners. With only a few exceptions, almost all studies we reviewed focused on anti-Black structural racism. This specific anti-Black focus is reflected in how the measures are calculated. For example, three-quarters (~75%) of the studies used measures of Black and White distribution in specific spatial units or used measures of Black–White disproportionality ratios (e.g., rates of access to employment for Black compared to White county residents) to examine structural racism.[13–35]

A handful of studies examined health inequities for Latinx people.[16,20,36–41] Other studies did not examine a Black–White health disparity and instead included only Black participants.[15,42–48] De-centering White people in analytical models allows these scholars to further examine heterogeneity in both exposure and the health effects of structural racism, and further examine critically why subgroups within a particular racialized community are less affected by structural racism than others.

Structural racism impacts all racialized groups, but the operationalization and measurement of structural racism impacting non-Black racialized groups is still limited. It is possible that some anti-Black structural racism measures could be universally applied to assess health inequities for Latinx, Asian and Pacific Islander, Native American, Alaska Native Americans, and other racial and ethnic groups. New structural racism measures may also need to be developed to specifically capture the unique historical and contemporary forms of structural racism that plague each racialized group in America. For example, given increasing evidence of xenophobia and anti-immigrant acts against East Asian people during the COVID-19 pandemic, special attention must be given to measuring anti-Asian structural racism, such as through travel restrictions. Even further specificity, such as measuring anti-Chinese structural racism, could be needed to accurately capture varying experiences of structural racism based on racial and ethnic identity.

Priority on Health in Early Life

Birth outcomes, early life, and mid-adult life were commonly examined in studies on structural racism and health, whereas end-of-life and older adults were less represented. In our review, we identified multiple studies that focused on maternal and infant health,[14,21,22,28-31,35,43,44,49-54] on populations of children,[20,42,48,] and on populations of adult age.[13,16-18,22,23,25-27,32,34,47,50,55-59] Because much of the work concerning structural racism is done using populations younger than retirement age, there is a gap in our understanding of how exposure to structural racism accumulates over time to influence health in later life, how structural racism uniquely manifests in later life, and what the implications of this exposure to structural racism are for researchers who study racial inequities for older adults, long-term care, and aging care.

Focusing on older adult populations is important to understanding the connections between historical and contemporary experiences with structural racism and current health inequities. In addition, our population is aging and requires increased use of long-term care services for older adults, and these services continue to be one of the most segregated institutions today.[60] This will be a critical gap to address as time goes on.

Emphasis on Segregation-driven Measures

Foundational literature on structural racism and health inequities highlights segregation as a key example of racist policies and practices that physically separate racialized communities from White communities.[4,61,62] Contemporary work also expands beyond primarily measuring racial residential segregation, using measures such as the index of dissimilarity, isolation index, and entropy index, with more recent scholarship adding a nuance of operationalizing and measuring structural racism as differential access to socioeconomic resources (e.g., high-quality school, employment, home loan) that are driven by residential segregation through the index of concentration at the extremes (ICE).

Residential segregation measures were used in almost half of the studies we reviewed, including the dissimilarity index,[13,22,23,25,27,35,48,59] isolation index,[22,29,37] and ICE.[14,19,22,24,26,28,39,43,51] Whereas the dissimilarity index captures the distribution of racialized groups within a defined space, ICE captures two dimensions, both racial residential segregation and income inequality, emphasizing the distribution of privilege (e.g., White race and high income) and disadvantage (e.g., Black race and low income) within a geographic area.

Neighborhood Is a Common Geographic Level of Analysis

Structural racism can be measured across a variety of geographic levels. Studies measure structural racism at the state level, [31,33,34,50,59] at the county level,[17,21,25,26,35,55] at the Metropolitan Statistical Area (MSA)/city level,[13,28,63] at a smaller neighborhood level (e.g., census tract/block, zip code, community-area),[14,15,19,20,26,32,33,42,48,49,56,58] and at the individual exposure level.[16,22] The use of neighborhood-based measures is grounded in the idea that where you live and spend the majority of your time matters. Most prominently, Krieger's (2012) ecosocial theory[64] and Geronimus's (1992) weathering effect[65] frameworks theorize that individuals embody racism and various forms of oppression around them. Over the life course, oppression can get "under the skin" and have negative impacts on the health of historically oppressed groups.

A critical decision when deciding on structural racism measures is what geographic unit to ground the measure in.[5] While studies of interpersonal and internalized racism use the individual as the unit of measurement, measures of structural racism are often estimated at the census tract, county, or state levels. Which level to use depends on the research question. It is important to emphasize that there is no gold standard recommendation for a geographic unit. Rather, as Chantarat and colleagues (2021),[13] and Riley (2019)[66] argue, structural racism should be measured at the spatial unit consistent with the mechanism that gives rise to it. For example, employment inequity, in which the corrupted job search process is the main mechanism driving structural racism in the labor market, should be measured at the labor markets spatial unit, like the community zone or MSA, which extends beyond the more specific neighborhood in which individuals live.[67]

From our review, structural racism is most commonly assessed at the county level. Some of the studies argue that their use of county measures is based on the notion that many racist laws are made at the county level. For example, preclearance coverage under the Voting Rights Act to monitor discrimination at the polls was issued at the county level, thus a logical study design could then examine counties covered and not covered by pre-clearance to examine the effect of this coverage on voting rates and health outcomes.[68] Yet other studies measured structural racism at the county level because of data access limitations, because only county-level population data (e.g., from the County Health Rankings database) are available to them to derive the measure.[69]

When thinking about geographic based measures of structural racism, one should also consider how those measures perform in urban areas compared to rural areas. Three studies examined how county-level structural racism measures performed in more rural versus more urban counties,[17,21,23] and determined that the association between structural racism measures and health varied by rural-urban county classification. Bell and colleagues (2020), and Vilda and colleagues (2020) found a non-significant association between structural racism and self-reported health[23] and infant mortality rates[21] in rural areas, but not urban areas. Given that there are comparatively fewer racialized residents in rural areas than White residents, the denominators for the rates for these groups are often unstable or non-calculable in rural areas compared to urban areas. Alternative measurement approaches may be needed to accurately capture the extent of structural racism and conclude if their impacts on health vary along the rural–urban continuum.

Development of Multi-level Spatial Units of Measurement

While the previous section detailed how structural racism can be measured at discrete geographic units, there are also opportunities to consider the intersections of how structural racism at the state level informs policies and practices at the county or neighborhood level. Understanding how policies are differentially applied downstream can provide insight into the mechanisms linking structural racism to health and where to intervene across various levels.

Racist policies and practices are implemented at different levels of government and institutions. However, few studies attempt to operationalize and measure structural racism across multiple geographic levels, such as neighborhoods nested in counties, or counties in states. All studies included in this report examined area-level measures of racism at only one level, such as the state, county, or MSA. None examined how structural racism across different levels interacts with one another. For example, does living in a state with high levels of incarceration have an effect above and beyond living in a city with lower incarceration rates? Is there even an interaction between different types of structural racism across levels? Do high levels of political disenfranchisement at the state level lead to higher levels of income inequality and educational inequality at the county level? How does that interaction influence health?

There are many multilevel questions that need to be investigated as we try to understand not only how structural racism manifests across levels and domains, but also how these manifestations impact health inequities.

A Need for Multidimensional Measures of Structural Racism

Across the studies we reviewed, about half examined only one domain of structural racism (e.g., residential segregation alone), while the other half considered the effect of multiple various domains (e.g., both residential segregation and education inequity in a single study) on the health of racialized communities. This is an increase in the number of studies incorporating multiple types of structural racism on health from the 2018 Groos and colleagues literature review.[9] Yet many studies used unidimensional measures of structural racism in housing and socioeconomic status, with one measure for each in a regression model, and, then, separately discussed the relative association of each to health. In other words, researchers showed the effect of each structural racism domain on health adjusted for the other, but did not actually interrogate how the two (or more) might be connected.

Only two articles characterized the interactions among various domains of structural racism to measure structural racism as a system-like determinant of health. These studies examined the joint effect (independent effect of each domain plus reinforcing effect across multiple domains) on health: Dougherty and colleagues (2019),[25] which established the county structural racism measure, and Chantarat and colleagues (2021),[13] which created the multidimensional measure of structural racism. Both studies consolidated multiple domains of structural racism together by employing a latent-variable approach commonly used among psychometricians for data reduction. Given a theoretical grounding that defines structural racism as a totality,[2] multidimensional measures like these pave a new way for population health scholars to more accurately examine the health impacts of structural racism. Both multidimensional measures have only been applied using one dataset each (Dougherty et al. used the Behavioral Risk Factor Surveillance System data; Chantarat et al. used COVID-19 vaccination data from New York City). Thus, more research is needed to validate these measures to ensure their external validity.

Counterfactual Simulation Analyses

Two studies we identified did not create structural racism measures, but instead used counterfactual simulation approaches to quantify the effects of structural racism on health inequities. Lundberg (2021)[16] estimated the effect of occupational segregation (i.e., racially patterned access to work and occupations) on racial inequity in disability that prevents workers from working or which limits the kind or amount of work.[22] Instead of deriving an exposure variable (i.e., x variable in regression equations such as a dissimilarity score) as most studies do, Lundberg used a counterfactual simulation approach to quantify gap-closing estimate. They estimated this by comparing the outcome of interest observed in the current labor market to the simulated one. A similar approach was used by Graetz and Esposito (2021),[26] who applied a counterfactual simulated approach to examine the extent to which changes in redlining grades influence later life expectancy and disparity in predominantly Black and White neighborhoods.

Using mathematical modeling to "measure" racial inequity is not new to the literature, yet the application of this approach to examine the role of structural racism on health inequities represents a new frontier. Given that mathematical models can be created using parameters from already published studies and require relatively limited data collection, this line of research should be explored in future studies. Further, while there are limitations to these models, they provide the opportunity to create a powerful alternative in which we can imagine how people might thrive when the oppressive forces of structural racism and White supremacy are removed.

Development of an Antiracism/Equity Measure

Only one measure sought to operationalize progress toward racial equity and antiracism: the National Equity Atlas.[63] The index consists of a composite score of nine measures divided into three domains: economic vitality (wages, unemployment, poverty), readiness (educational attainment, disconnected youth, school poverty), and connectedness (air pollution exposure, commute time, housing burden). Instead of measuring the gap between racial groups as the metric, the racial equity index evaluates how close the experiences of all racial groups are to the population average. Given that the goal of antiracism research and policy is dismantling the system of oppression to achieve racial equity in all aspects of life, equity/antiracism measures have the potential to be used as a progress tracking tool to examine the effectiveness of interventions. Though limited attention has been given to creating positive progress measures, future research should aim to capture progress in addition to documenting problems.

Barnraising Conversations: Key Takeaways

The 2022 Barnraising event on measuring structural racism encompassed a remarkably productive one and a half days. From the conversations during the Barnraising working groups, the participants converged upon key recommendations and next steps. Six themes emerged from these discussions that should guide future research and funding priorities.

Measuring Structural Racism is Difficult

The group recognized that there is not a gold-standard measure for every structural racism domain or for every group affected or across time—and likely never will be. While the population health community works continuously to improve structural racism measures, the tools that we have are incomplete, yielding only a partial picture of structural racism. For those working to dismantle structural racism, not having an agreed-upon, validated approach to use in research could be discouraging. Yet all participants agreed that some progress is better than none, and that we "should not let perfect be the enemy of good."

For example, the novel multidimensional measure of structural racism by Chantarat and colleagues[13] captures cross-sectionally how residential segregation, inequities in education, employment, income, and homeownership jointly impact health. While this methodological leap allows researchers to better understand the mechanistic relationship between structural racism and health inequities, this cross-sectional measure does not capture the changing/morphing of structural racism over time. Despite these limitations, these methodological advances in measuring structural racism are still important steps forward in the work of antiracism.

In addition to new measures, new tools are also required to create more complete measures of structural racism. As structural racism operates as a system, a system-based approach could better approximate structural racism than siloed individual measures.[1,4,6] Multidisciplinary knowledge from systems-science-focused fields such as engineering could be useful in operationalizing and measuring structural racism as a multidimensional determinant of health.[5,10] An implementation science approach called the Consolidated Framework for Implementation Research (CFIR) was suggested as a potential framework to guide the future development of structural racism measures.[70]

Workshop participants also agreed that since structural racism manifests differently across the life course and across time, researchers must develop a "framework" that is adaptable for different research questions rather than focusing on creating specific measures that can be used in all scenarios.

Measuring Equity/Antiracism

Beyond capturing the harms of structural racism, the group discussed how to measure equity, joy, and resilience. How do communities survive and thrive despite the experiences and pervasiveness of structural racism? What roles do joy and resilience play for historical and contemporary racialized communities? In our review, we identified one measure of equity called the racial equity index (see Development of an Antiracism/Equity Measure above).[63] Future research should explore how to measure alternative structures created by groups experiencing oppression, such as mutual aid networks or community-based organizations, and how their existence buffers the impact of structural racism on health.

The group agreed that when measuring structural racism, it is critical for researchers to be cognizant of the way in which research traditions can reinforce White supremacy. Researchers must consider our own biases and how our perspectives have been shaped by White supremacy, and they must acknowledge the historical and contemporary harm perpetuated against racialized communities by academic and medical institutions. Critically, researchers must also ensure our questions and solutions represent the *community's* perspectives, definitions of health and well-being, and collective vision—*not* the academy's or anyone else's.

Causal Inference versus Causal Assumption

Antiracism researchers are often required to respond to questions and concerns regarding causality—specifically, whether their study demonstrates a causal relationship between structural racism and the health outcome they studied. From the statistical and econometric points of view, statistical causal inference can be made if the exposure of interest (structural racism, in our case) is randomized, all confounders are controlled for, and the appropriate temporality between exposure and outcomes of interest is established.

In structural racism and health research, satisfying all these criteria for causal inference is difficult, if not impossible. We cannot randomize one group of people to live in a racially oppressed society while the other group lives in an equitable society in the real world. So, in the traditional causal-inference framework, only associations, not causal relationships, can be established. Participants pushed back on this limiting traditional framework, bringing up two key counterpoints. First, the way in which scholars perceive "causal inference" is based on the seminal writing of a few White scholars, namely Judea Pearl, Jamie Robins, and Miguel Hernan.[71–73] The traditional canon of causal inference is not aligned with the advancement of inquiry as to how structural racism affects health. Thus, alternative approaches are needed. Second, the literature has failed to fully attribute persistent racial health inequities to alternative theoretical causes such as socioeconomic conditions and access to resources. It is theoretically and ethically appropriate to assume that racial health inequities are fundamentally caused by structural racism.

Health Equity Tourism

The group recognized that many researchers are becoming interested in structural racism research, following a significant increase from journals and funding organizations issuing requests for proposals on this topic. As Dr. Elle Lett and colleagues[74] noted, the increased attention to structural racism research could lead to an influx of health equity tourism, characterized as "the process of previously unengaged investigators pivoting into health equity research, without developing the necessary scientific expertise for high-quality work."[74] While more research is certainly needed, the group wanted to exercise caution to ensure funding priorities go to authentic antiracism research that is conceptualized and led by those dedicated to dismantling White supremacy.

For funders who have recently shifted their funding priority to antiracism research, it is just as critical to have appropriate experts who can critically review and comment on incoming proposals. Making blanket funding available for this line of work is not enough, as misdirected resources could exacerbate harm and exploitation of structural racism on racialized communities. In addition to incorporating expert reviewers, funders should also bolster their own capacity to provide guidance for reviewers who may not be directly familiar with structural racism scholarship. Funders have the unique privilege of protecting against the harms of health equity tourism by attending to the principles put forth by Lett and colleagues.[74]

Community-engaged Research to Improve Measurement

Throughout the Barnraising, a continual theme was including the community. However, it was noted through the discussions that in order to move forward with this, we must be clear about how we are *defining* community. Importantly, many antiracism researchers themselves *are* members of a community that is disproportionately impacted by structural racism. While this report focuses solely on quantitative measures, qualitative methods can uniquely contribute to operationalization and measurement. As stated in Hardeman and colleagues (2022), "Qualitative research also plays a critical role in the understanding of structural racism and its impact on health. Indeed, qualitative data provide rich information about the lived experience of structural racism by allowing people closest to the reality of structural racism to describe how racism affects their lives."[5]

Interviews, focus groups, ethnographies, and participant observation can shape our understanding of how different domains of structural racism interact. Perhaps domains should be weighted to account for this differential impact. Further, structural racism does not manifest in the same way across the life course.[75,76] Through conversations and inclusion of community voices, researchers can identify at which time points different forms of structural racism have the greatest impacts upon health.

The ultimate goal of this work is to dismantle structural racism to achieve health equity. That work cannot be done without including those harmed by structural racism, so that they can help to reimagine a more equitable future.

Future Steps

This chapter offers critical key steps in the advancement of the field around operationalizing and measuring structural racism. For funders, these suggestions are the types of innovative studies that will push the field forward in the goal of dismantling structural racism and achieving racial equity through policy solutions. A summary of guiding questions for funders can be found in Table 4.1.

First, the most commonly used measures were the dissimilarity index, disproportionality index, and index of concentration at the extremes. These are all used to measure residential segregation. We must expand the types of structural racism we are measuring beyond residential segregation. Compared to the review published in 2018,[9] there is now more diversity in the domains of structural racism being measured. In addition to residential segregation, inequities in education, employment, homeownership, and home loan access, new measures of racial inequities in incarceration, political participation, reparations, and occupational mobility are being used. While most measures still rely on population estimates from sources like the ACS (extracted from a harmonized database like IPUMS), HMDA, and County Health Ranking database, newly released databases like the Vera Institute of Justice,[77] Pew Research Center,[78] Global Burden of Disease Collaboration Network,[79] Eviction Lab,[80] National Conference of State

Table 4.1 Guiding questions for funders based on the next steps suggested in this report

---

What data can we use and how can it be improved?

A data repository with measures of many domains of structural racism, across time, and across geographic contexts that can be connected to health outcomes is needed to allow for more complex research to occur. Research that begins this linking process and identifies new sources of structural racism data is vital and necessary.

When should structural racism be measured? How can we examine the links between historic and contemporary forms of structural racism?

Time is an important component of structural racism research. We should consider carefully how historic forms of structural racism manifest today to impact health and prioritize studies that address these questions.

How can we measure structural racism in a more holistic manner?

As we continue to operationalize structural racism, we must keep in mind that measures will be good, but not perfect. New methods and models will be developed that will improve upon current and future approaches, but we must not be discouraged by their lack of precision today.

Multidimensional measures should be prioritized which examine how multiple domains of structural racism interact to impact health. Unidimensional measures should still be developed, as there are many domains of structural racism that we are just beginning to measure (e.g., voter suppression, police violence), and these should also be funded, but multidimensional measures are also needed to fully understand how structural racism operates as a system to influence health.

How is community being defined and represented? How is the community benefiting from this research?

---

continued

Table 4.1 *continued*

Are members of the community on a research advisory board? Are community voices being used to inform the study? Will the research help or harm the community?

Who is doing the research and who should be funded?
Does funding this project contribute to the threat of health equity tourism?

How are reviewers chosen? What expertise and lived experience do they bring as reviewers?

Legislatures,[81] and the Stanford Open Policing Project[82] are resources for operationalizing and measuring structural racism. Researchers interested in studying multiple domains of structural racism still need to separately extract data from multiple databases. These steps are cumbersome and time-consuming, especially for individuals outside the academic setting who may not have the skill set and resources to do so.

Next Steps

- **Short term:** A significant shift in the data infrastructure aimed at measuring structural racism will take time. In the interim, research institutions or organizations should seek to support scholars and activists who have shown dedication and expertise, and have experienced the consequences of structural racism in their lives and communities—a practice which would help protect against health equity tourism. This support could take the form of providing free data management, consultation, and analytic services to such scholars.

- **Long term:** In the long run, creating a data repository linking all databases mentioned above together will make the extraction of data needed to create structural racism measures easier for those interested in advancing this line of work.

Second, many measures of structural racism are contemporary, examining structural racism in the twenty-first century, with some stretching back to the 1950s and 1960s to examine the impact of Civil Rights advances on health. Yet few measures of structural racism focus on the time period after Emancipation but before Jim Crow. More historical data is needed to understand how historic oppression impacts population health today. We did not identify any study between 2019 and 2021 that measures structural racism with historical data. However, one study published in 2015 found that places with slavery in the 1860s continue to have lower rates of voting to this day.[68] Further, structural racism evolves over time; when one form of structural racism is stopped or altered through policy, new iterations develop to achieve the same means of marginalization and oppression. For example, the modern police force developed from slave patrols; voter identification laws and poll closures are a descendent of literacy tests and poll taxes; and forced labor under incarceration developed from slavery. Identifying manifestations of structural racism across historic and contemporary periods will yield further understanding of how structural racism evolves and transforms, and influences the health of racialized communities over time.

Next Steps

- **Short term:** More research that uses historical data is needed to understand how historic structural racism influences contemporary structural racism and contemporary health inequities. Furthermore, we need historical data to track this evolution, expansion, and contraction across domains. In seeing this story over centuries, we can also identify which interventions were most successful and see how structural racism evolves when facing different barriers. This can inform future interventions and provide a better understanding of how to dismantle structural racism.
- **Long term:** These historical measures of structural racism must be included in the aforementioned data repository.

Third, just as structural racism can mutate overtime, the methods that are being used to measure it should evolve as well. As we observed, the standard statistical approach is to use one or two unidimensional measures of structural racism in a regression model, yet this practice is incomplete as it does not allow for the joint effect of different domains of structural racism to be measured. As structural racism operates as a system, it follows that a systems approach is necessary to measure its impact on health. Across other disciplines, such as engineering, systems-science approaches have been applied and could be adapted as a new method for racism research. Others have incorporated methods from other social science disciplines, such as mathematical models, latent class, and factor models. Two studies challenge the standard approach through their application of a latent-construct approach to operationalize and measure structural racism as a multidimensional determinant of health.[25,67] This approach represents a novel and critical leap toward accurately measuring structural racism and its many complexities. Yet the external validity for both of these newly proposed measures and whether their effectiveness in capturing structural racism (i.e., do they both capture the same things) has not been tested. Prioritizing funding of more novel approaches is necessary to move the field forward.

Next Steps

Future measures should attempt to operationalize the joint effect across structural racism domains, to consider how different forms of structural racism and other forms of structural oppression (e.g., structural sexism, classism) work in tandem to impact health. This could look like the measure of structural intersectionality put forth by Homan and colleagues. (2021). Funding for the external validation (e.g., using the measure with other datasets) and improvement of these multidimensional measures should also be prioritized.

Fourth, we must focus on who creates the knowledge as much as the approach we used to create it. Researchers who have dedicated their careers to advancing antiracism research and policy and community members affected by structural racism must lead all efforts to create antiracism knowledge and policy solutions. As part of this consideration, funders and reviewers must also be wary of the recent increase of health equity tourists in structural racism research—those who may be motivated by new streams of funding to support this line of work but have limited expertise in antiracism content and methodological expertise.[74] Further, who is reviewing grants and proposals is important to consider. Reviewers must reflect the communities impacted by the proposed research and possess the requisite expertise and antiracist lens.

Next Steps

To minimize health equity tourism, funders must reexamine the way in which proposals are scored and who scores the proposal. Priority should be given to research led or co-led by non-academic organizations that have a rich knowledge of how structural racism harms health and work closely with the community to dismantle structural racism. An example of this kind of program is the RWJF Interdisciplinary Research Leaders,[69] which advances the co-creation of sustainable racial health policy solutions in the community.

Operationalizing structural racism and funding structural racism research is a key path toward understanding and dismantling the link between structural racism and health inequities. Our analysis of the state of the literature on measures of structural racism in the past three years in the public health literature can serve as a resource in shaping an antiracist path forward for funders.

Appendices

Appendix I: Improving the Measurement of Structural Racism Barnraising daily agenda

Improving the Measurement of Structural Racism Barnraising
Co-hosted by the Minnesota Population Center (MPC) and the Center for Antiracism Research for Health Equity (CARHE)

Monday, March 14th
Welcome and Mingle
9:00–9:30 a.m. Central Time|120 Elmer L. Andersen Library, University of Minnesota Twin Cities Campus - West Bank

Participants trickle into the event space. There will be time to get your name tags and mingle with people. Coffee, water, and tea will be provided along with fruit and small snacks.

For our out-of-town guests, J'Mag Karbeah will meet you at the Courtyard Marriott Lobby at 9:00 a.m. to walk you over to the venue (approximately a 5 minute walk).

Our Charge to the Group by Dr. Rachel Hardeman
9:30–10:30 a.m. Central Time|120 Elmer L. Andersen Library

We'll do a welcome, provide an overview of the event structure, and lay the groundwork for the next day and a half.

15 Minute Break
Beverages will be provided.

Expert Panel Discussion
Monday, March 14th|10:45 a.m.–12:00 p.m. Central Time
120 Elmer L. Andersen Library and available on Zoom

Our invited panelists discuss where they see the needs and where progress can be made. There will also be time for open discussion.

Moderator: Rachel Hardeman, PhD, MPH, Director of the Center for Antiracism Research for Health Equity at the University of Minnesota

Panelists:
Paris Adkins-Jackson, PhD, MPH, Research Associate at Johns Hopkins University
Roland Thorpe Jr., PhD, MS, Co-Director of DRPH Concentration in Health, Equity, and Social Justice Professor at Johns Hopkins Bloomberg School of Public Health
Tyson Brown, PhD, Director of the Center on Health & Society and Associate Professor of Sociology at Duke University

Lunch Mixer
12:00 p.m.–1:00 p.m. Central Time|120 Elmer L. Andersen Library,

Box lunches and beverages will be provided. This is a time for informal conversation and a chance to move and mingle.

15 Minute Break

Working Group Meeting 1
1:15–2:30 p.m. Central Time
"How can IPUMS data help us measure the intersectionality of structural racism?" facilitated by Kari Williams.
"What do community stakeholders need from measures of structural racism?" facilitated by Miamon Queeglay and J'Mag Karbeah.

Half of the group will be in <u>120 Elmer L. Andersen Library</u> the other half will be in the Institute for Social Research and Data Innovation seminar room in <u>Willey Hall</u>.

15 Minute Break

Working Group Meeting 2
2:45–4:00 p.m. Central Time
"How do we accurately measure structural racism?" facilitated by Dr. Roland Thorpe and Dr. Bert Chantarat.

"What data/datasets do we need to measure structural racism?" facilitated by Dr. Paris Adkins-Jackson and Dr. Rachel Hardeman.

Half of the group will be in <u>120 Elmer L. Andersen Library</u> the other half will be in the Institute for Social Research and Data Innovation seminar room in <u>Willey Hall</u>.

See the other attached document to see what working group you have been assigned to. We will have people available to walk the groups from one venue to the other.

Tuesday, March 15th
For our out-of-town guests, <u>Bert Chantarat</u> will meet you at the <u>Courtyard Marriott</u> Lobby at 8:45 a.m. to walk you over to the venue (approximately a 5 minute walk).

Working Group Report and Discussion, facilitated by Keelia Silvis
9:00 a.m.–11:15 a.m. Central Time| Institute for Social Research and Data Innovation seminar room in 50 <u>Willey Hall</u> and on <u>Zoom</u>

The small working groups report back to the larger group and we discuss all together what ideas, thoughts, and solutions they came up with.

Coffee, water, and tea will be provided along with fruit and small snacks.

15 Minute Break

Next Steps/Wrap Up, facilitated by Dr. Rachel Hardeman
11:30 a.m.–12:00 p.m. Central Time| Institute for Social Research and Data Innovation seminar room in 50 <u>Willey Hall</u>

Time to discuss what our next steps will be and where we go from here given what we've discussed and learned.

Final Conversation Lunch
12:00–1:00 p.m. Central Time| Institute for Social Research and Data Innovation seminar room in 50 <u>Willey Hall</u>

Appendix II: Table 4.1 Common structural racism measures

Structural racism measure	Data source(s)	Methodology in estimation
Residential Dissimilarity Index	American Community Survey	$D = \frac{1}{2} \sum_{i=1}^{n} \left(\frac{a_i}{A} - \frac{b_i}{B} \right)$ Where: a_i = the population of group A in the ith area, e.g., census tract A = the total population in group A in the large geographic entity for which the index of dissimilarity is being calculated. b_i = the population of group B in the ith area B = the total population in group B in the large geographic entity for which the index of dissimilarity is being calculated. n = number of large geographic entities. (Massey DS, Denton NA. The Dimensions of Residential Segregation. *Social Forces.* 1988;67(2):281–315.)

Structural racism measure	Data source(s)	Methodology in estimation
Isolation index	US Census of Population and Housing	$IoI = \sum_{i=1}^{n} \left[\left(\frac{x_i}{X} \right) \left(\frac{y_i}{t_i} \right) \right]$ Where: n = the number of areas (census tracts) in the metropolitan area, ranked smallest to largest by land area x_i = the minority population of area i X = the sum of all xi (the total minority population) t_i = the total population of area i (Massey DS, Denton NA. The Dimensions of Residential Segregation. *Social Forces.* 1988;67(2):281–315.)
Index of Concentration at the Extremes (ICE)	American Community Survey (for census tract measure) Elementary/ Secondary Information System (for school district measure)	Can be used for race, income, and race+income, in various geographic unit (e.g., census tract, school district) $ICE = \frac{A-P}{T}$ Where: A = number of White households with income of $100,000 or higher (privileged group) P = number of Black households with income lower than $25,000 (deprived group) T = total number of Black and White households in the PUMA ICE ranges from −1 (all households are in the deprived group) to 1 (all households are in the privileged group). (Feldman JM, Waterman PD, Coull BA, Krieger N. Spatial social polarization: Using the index of concentration at the extremes jointly for income and race/ethnicity to analyse risk of hypertension. *Journal of Epidemiology and Community Health.* 2015;69(12):1199–1207. Massey DS. The prodigal paradigm returns: Ecology comes back to sociology. *Does It Take Village.* 2001:41–48.)

continued

continued

Structural racism measure	Data source(s)	Methodology in estimation
Black-white spatial exposure score (P*)	American Community Survey	$$_b(P^*)_w = \int_{q \in R} \frac{\tau_{qb}}{T_b} \pi_{qw} dq$$ Where: π_{qw} = weighted proportion of White individuals within census tract q's local environment T_b = total number of Black individuals within county T_{qb} = total number of Black individuals within census tract q = each census tract (Reardon SF, O'Sullivan D. Measures of spatial segregation. Sociol Methodol Wiley Online Library. 2004;34:121–162.)
Spatial Information Theory Index (H)	American Community Survey	$$H = 1 - \frac{\int_{q \in R}(\tau_q x\, E_q)dq}{TxE}$$ Where: E = overall county entropy of the total population calculated as $$\sum_m (proportion\ of\ m\ in\ county)\ x\ logM$$ (*proportion of m in county*) τ_q = population density at q T = total population in county (Reardon SF, O'Sullivan D. Measures of spatial segregation. Sociology Methodology. 2004;34:121–162.)
Index of Spatial Proximity (ISP)	American Community Survey	$$ISP = \frac{XP_{xx} - YP_{yy}}{TP_{tt}}$$ Where: $$P_{gg} = \sum_{i=1}^{n} \sum_{j=1}^{n} \frac{(g_i g_c c_{ij})}{G^2}$$ and (g,G) = (x,X), (y,Y), (t,T) n = number of areas in the metropolitan areas, ranked smallest to largest by land area x_i = the minority population of area i X = the sum of all x_i y_i = the majority population of area i Y = the sum of all y_i ti = the total population of area i T = the sum of all t_i P = the ratio of X to T

Structural racism measure	Data source(s)	Methodology in estimation
		(White MJ, The measurement of spatial segregation. *American Journal of Sociology.* 1983;88(5):1008–1018.)
Black-white (or white-Black) Dispropor-tionality Ratios	American Community Survey(ACS)	Ratios span measures of socioeconomic status, political participation, ambulatory care, and incarceration rates.
	Robert Wood Johnson Foundation County Health Rankings	Ratio = rate for Black people/rate for White people
	Vera Institute of Justice (consolidation of data from the US Department of Justice Bureau of Justice Statistics Census of Jails and the Annual Survey of Jails, National Prisoner Statistics)	
Multidimen-sional Measure of Structural Racism	American Community Survey	Multidimensional typologies derived from five structural racism measures: Black–White residential segregation (measured with a dissimilarity index) White–Black education inequity White–Black employment inequity White–Black homeownership Income equity (measured by the index of concentration at the extremes).
		Multidimensional typologies are identified with the latent class analysis model.
		(Chantarat T, Van Riper DC, Hardeman RR. The intricacy of structural racism measurement: A pilot development of a latent-class multidimensional measure. *eClinicalMedicine.* 2021;40:101092. doi:10.1016/j.eclinm.2021.101092.)
State Racism Index	American Community Survey	Average of Segregation Index, Incarceration Index, Education Index, Economic Index, and Employment Index—all measured at the state level. See Siegel et al. (2021, Table 2) for the equations for all the measures.
	Vera Institute of Justice Jail Incarceration	

continued

continued

Structural racism measure	Data source(s)	Methodology in estimation
		(Siegel M, Critchfield-Jain I, Boykin M, Owens A, Muratore R, Nunn T, Oh J. Racial/ethnic disparities in state-level COVID-19 vaccination rates and their association with structural racism. *Journal of Racial and Ethnic Health Disparities.* Published online October 28, 2021. doi:10.1007/s40615-021-01173-7.)
Structural Intersection-ality (state-level)	US Census Bureau Data, Bureau of Labor Statistics Center for American women and Politics Guttmacher Institute	Summation of the score from the following measures: White–Black Ratio of incarceration Blacks' disproportionate level of Disenfranchisement White–Black Ratio of proportion with a bachelor's degree White–Black Ratio of unemployed rate White–Black Ratio of poverty rate White–Black Ratio of proportion who are homeowners White–Black Ratio of proportion who voted in 2008 Level of black's political underrepresentation in state legislatures State-level dissimilarity index (Black-white) of residential segregation. (Homan P, Brown TH, King B. Structural intersectionality as a new direction for health disparities research. *Journal of Health and Social Behavior.* 2021;62(3):350–370. doi:10.1177/00221465211032947.)
County Structural Racism	Census of Jail Inmates Department of Education Common Core of Data American Community Survey Dartmouth Atlas of Health Care	A factor score from confirmatory factor analysis combining the following measures: Black–White jail incarceration ratio White–Black high school graduation ratio School dissimilarity index Black–White poverty ratio Black–White ratio of proportion of Medicare beneficiaries discharged from a hospital for an ambulatory care sensitive condition

Structural racism measure	Data source(s)	Methodology in estimation
		White–Black ratio of average annual proportion of Medicare enrollees having at least one ambulatory visit to a primary care clinician H entropy index (Dougherty GB, Golden SH, Gross AL, Colantuoni E, Dean LT. Measuring structural racism and its association with BMI. *American Journal of Preventive Medicine.* 2020;59(4):530–537. doi:10.1016/j.amepre.2020.05.019.)
County Structural Racism score	American Community Survey (ACS) Vera Institute of Justice Jail Incarceration data	Summation of three dichotomizing county-level structural racism measures. For each measure, the value higher than the 75th percentile of all US counties is considered "high" (score 1), or "low" (score 0) otherwise. The three structural racism measures that make up the county structural racism score are: White–Black ratio in proportions of the population age 25 years and older with a bachelor's degree or higher White–Black ratio in median household income Black–White ratio in jail incarceration (Vilda D, Hardeman R, Dyer L, Theall KP, Wallace, M. Structural racism, racial inequities and urban rural differences in infant mortality in the US. *Journal of Epidemiology and Community Health.* 2021;75(8):788–793. doi:10.1136/jech-2020-214260.)
Overall Measure of State Structural Racism	US Decennial Census Current Population Survey US Department of Justice, Bureau of Justice Statistics data	Summation of eight dichotomized state-level structural racism measures. For each measure, the value higher than the median of all US states is considered "high" (score 1), or "low" (score 0) otherwise. The eight structural racism measures that make up the state structural racism score are: Black–White ratio in proportions of the population who earned a bachelor's degrees or higher

continued

continued

Structural racism measure	Data source(s)	Methodology in estimation
		Black–White ratio in proportions of the population who registered to vote
		Black–White ratio in proportions of the population who voted
		Black–White ratio in proportions of the population who are in civilian labor force
		Black–White ratio in proportions of the population who are employed
		Black–White ratio in proportions of the population who hold executive position
		Black–White ratio in proportions of the population who have professional specialty
		Black–White incarceration ratio (Lukachko A, Hatzenbuehler ML, Keyes KM. Structural racism and myocardial infarction in the United States. *Social Science & Medicine*. 2014;103:4250. doi:10.1016/j.socscimed.2013.07.021.
		Volpe VV, Schorpp KM, Cacace SC, Benson GP, Banos NC. State- and provider-level racism and health care in the U.S. *American Journal of Preventive Medicine*. 2021;61(3):338–347. doi:10.1016/j.amepre.2021.03.008.)
Dual mortgage market political economies measures	Project of Human Development in Chicago Neighborhoods Home Mortgage Disclosure Act Neighborhood Change Database	A set of four measures that includes: Neighborhood credit refusals: Ratio of the rate of access to the mortgage market for ethnoracially marginalized applicants (Blacks and Latinx) to the rate for ethnoracially privileged applicants (Whites) for specific area Racialized credit refusals: Ratio of the rate of access to the mortgage market for ethnoracially marginalized applicants (Blacks and Latinx) to the rate for ethnoracially privileged applicants (Whites) across areas Neighborhood credit privateness: Ratio of the rate of the federal oversight of originated loans for ethnoracially marginalized applicants (Blacks and Latinx) to the rate for ethnoracially privileged applicants (Whites) for specific area

Structural racism measure	Data source(s)	Methodology in estimation
		Racialized credit privateness: Ratio of the rate of the federal oversight of originated loans for ethnoracially marginalized applicants (Blacks and Latinx) to the rate for ethnoracially privileged applicants (Whites) across areas (Sewell, AA. Political economies of acute childhood illnesses: measuring structural racism as mesolevel mortgage market risks. *Ethnicity & Disease*. 2021;31, no. Suppl 1:319–332. https://pubmed.ncbi.nlm.nih.gov/34045834/.)
HOLC-assessed redlining measure	Home Owners' Loan Corporation (HOLC) Data Richmond Mapping Project	1930s HOLC neighborhood grading map (Nelson R, Winling L, Marciano R, Connolly N. *Mapping inequality*. n.d. Accessed July 22, 2021. https://dsl.richmond.edu/panorama/redlining/.)
Parish-level jail incarceration prevalence among black individuals	Vera Institute of Justice (jail incarceration data)	Count of Black individuals aged 16 to 64 in jail per 1,000 Black non-incarcerated residents (Dyer L, Hardeman R, Vilda D, Theall K, Wallace M. Mass incarceration and public health: The association between black jail incarceration and adverse birth outcomes among black women in Louisiana." *BMC Pregnancy and Childbirth*. 2019;19(1):525. doi:10.1186/s12884-019-2690-z.)
Racialized event (i.e. Flint Water Crisis)	N/A	Vicarious exposure to structural racism-related events. Residency in the areas after the racialized event occurs is treated as an exposure in a quasi-experimental model (e.g., difference-in-difference). (Allgood, KL. Equal protection under the law: *The measurement of structural racism and health disparities*. [PhD, University of Michigan; 2021]. https://www.proquest.com/docview/2592539075/abstract/2AC8B453EAA94018PQ/3.)
Number of Police Encounters	AddHealth	Response to a survey question, "How many times have you been stopped or detained by the police for questioning about your activities? Don't count minor traffic violations."

continued

continued

Structural racism measure	Data source(s)	Methodology in estimation
		This five-level categorical variable includes response options which range from 0 (never) to 6 or more times.
		(Allgood, KL. Equal protection under the law: The measurement of structural racism and health disparities. [PhD, University of Michigan; 2021]. https://www.proquest.com/docview/2592539075/abstract/2AC8B453EAA94018PQ/3.)
Economic Mobility Gap	Opportunity Atlas	Intergenerational gap in upward economic mobility conditional on parental income for Black and White adults.
		For details, see Chetty et al. *The opportunity atlas: Mapping the childhood roots of social mobility.* NBER working paper 25147. Cambridge, MA: National Bureau of Economic Research, 2019.
Racial Opportunity Gap	Opportunity Insights Data Library	The difference in the average national income percentile ranking in adulthood achieved between white and black individuals in the same county born to parents at the 25th percentile of the national income distribution
		(O'Brien R, Neman T, Seltzer N, Evans L, Venkataramani A. Structural racism, economic opportunity and racial health disparities: Evidence from U.S. counties. *SSM—Population Health.* 2020;11:100564. doi:10.1016/j.ssmph.2020.100564.)
County-level urban renewal projects	Richmond Renewing Project	The average of urban renewal projects in the counties overlapping with each Census tract.
		(Graetz N, Esposito M. Historical redlining and contemporary racial disparities in neighborhood life expectancy. Published online October 20, 2021. doi:10.31235/osf.io/q9gbx.)
Tract-level home values	Zillow Home Value Index	See detailed description at https://www.zillow.com/research/zhvi-methodology-2019-highlights-26221/
		(Graetz N, Esposito M. Historical redlining and contemporary racial disparities in neighborhood life expectancy. Published online October 20, 2021. doi:10.31235/osf.io/q9gbx.)

Structural racism measure	Data source(s)	Methodology in estimation
Racial equity index	National Equity Atlas	Utilizes an inclusion score and a prosperity score, also use formula for index of disparity
		(For National Equity Atlas, see: Treuhaft S, Langston A, Scoggins J, Lee J, Pastor M. The Racial Equity Index: A new data tool to drive local efforts to dismantle structural racism. *National Equity Atlas.* July 23, 2020. https://nationalequityatlas.org/research/index-findings.
		For index of disparity, see: Pearcy J, Keppel K. A summary measure of health disparity. *Public Health Reports.* 1974;117:273–280. Doi:10.1016/S0033-3549(04)50161-9.)

References

1. Gee GC, Hicken MT. Structural Racism: The Rules and Relations of Inequity. *Ethnicity & Disease.* 2021;31(Suppl 1):293–300. doi: 10.18865/ed.31.S1.293
2. Bailey ZD, Krieger N, Agénor M, Graves J, Linos N, Bassett MT. Structural racism and health inequities in the USA: Evidence and interventions. *The Lancet.* 2017;389(10077):1453–1463. doi:10.1016/S0140-6736(17)30569-X
3. Aspen Institute. We need a new social contract to undo a system of white supremacy. *The Aspen Institute.* July 9, 2020. https://www.aspeninstitute.org/blog-posts/undo-a-system-of-white-supremacy/.
4. Reskin B. The race discrimination system. *Annual Review of Sociology.* 2012;38(1):17–35. doi:10.1146/annurev-soc-071811-145508
5. Hardeman RR, Homan PA, Chantarat T, Davis BA, Brown TH. Improving the measurement of structural racism to achieve antiracist health policy. *Health Affairs.* 2022;41(2):179–186. doi:10.1377/hlthaff.2021.01489
6. Bonilla-Silva E. Rethinking racism: Toward a structural interpretation. *American Sociological Review.* 1997;62(3):465–480. doi:10.2307/2657316
7. Jones CP. Levels of racism: A theoretic framework and a gardener's tale. *American Journal of Public Health.* 2000;90(8):1212–1215.
8. Williams DR, Lawrence JA, Davis BA. Racism and health: Evidence and needed research. *Annual Review of Public Health.* 2019;40(1):105–125. doi:10.1146/annurev-publhealth-040218-043750
9. Groos M, Theall K, Wallace M, Hardeman R. Measuring inequity: a systematic review of methods used to quantify structural racism. *The Journal of Health Disparities Research and Practice.* 2018;11:190–206.
10. Hardeman RR, Medina EM, Boyd RW. Stolen breaths. *New England Journal of Medicine.* 2020;383(3):197–199. doi:10.1056/NEJMp2021072
11. Adkins-Jackson PB, Chantarat T, Bailey ZD, Ponce NA. Measuring structural racism: A guide for epidemiologists and other health researchers. *American Journal of Epidemiology.* September 25, 2021:kwab239. doi:10.1093/aje/kwab239

12. Taylor J, Pagliari C. Comprehensive scoping review of health research using social media data. *British Medical Journal Open*. 2018;8(12):e022931. doi:10.1136/bmjopen-2018-022931

13. Chantarat T, Van Riper DC, Hardeman RR. The intricacy of structural racism measurement: A pilot development of a latent-class multidimensional measure. *eClinicalMedicine*. 2021;40:101092. doi:10.1016/j.eclinm.2021.101092

14. Chambers BD, Baer RJ, McLemore MR, Jelliffe-Pawlowski LL. Using index of concentration at the extremes as indicators of structural racism to evaluate the association with preterm birth and infant mortality—California, 2011–2012. *Journal of Urban Health*. 2019;96(2):159–170. doi:10.1007/s11524-018-0272-4

15. Matoba N, Suprenant S, Rankin K, Yu H, Collins JW. Mortgage discrimination and preterm birth among African American women: An exploratory study. *Health & Place*. 2019;59:1. doi:10.1016/j.healthplace.2019.102193

16. Lundberg I. Quantifying the contribution of occupational segregation to racial disparities in health: A gap-closing perspective. Published online April 28, 2021. doi:10.31235/osf.io/x9evk

17. Bell C, Kerr J, Young J. Associations between Obesity, Obesogenic Environments, and Structural Racism Vary by County-Level Racial Composition. *International Journal of Environmental Research and Public Health*. 2019;16(5):861. doi:10.3390/ijerph16050861

18. O'Brien R, Neman T, Seltzer N, Evans L, Venkataramani A. Structural racism, economic opportunity and racial health disparities: Evidence from U.S. counties. *SSM—Population Health*. 2020;11:100564. doi:10.1016/j.ssmph.2020.100564

19. Dyer L, Chambers BD, Crear-Perry J, Theall KP, Wallace M. The index of concentration at the extremes (ICE) and pregnancy-associated mortality in Louisiana, 2016–2017. *Maternal and Child Health Journal*. June 19, 2021. doi:10.1007/s10995-021-03189-1

20. Sewell AA. Political Economies of Acute Childhood Illnesses: Measuring Structural Racism as Mesolevel Mortgage Market Risks. *Ethnicity & Disease*. May 20, 2021;31(Suppl 1):319–332. doi: 10.18865/ed.31.S1.319

21. Vilda D, Hardeman R, Dyer L, Theall KP, Wallace M. Structural racism, racial inequities and urban–rural differences in infant mortality in the US. *Journal of Epidemiology and Community Health*. 2021;75(8):788–793. doi:10.1136/jech-2020-214260

22. Allgood KL. *Equal protection under the law: The measurement of structural racism and health disparities*. [PhD, University of Michigan; 2021]. https://www.proquest.com/pqdtglobal/docview/2592539075/abstract/6523815FD2346F0PQ/3.

23. Bell CN, Owens-Young JL. Self-rated health and structural racism indicated by county-level racial inequalities in socioeconomic status: The role of urban-rural classification. *Journal of Urban Health*. 2020;97(1):52–61. doi:10.1007/s11524-019-00389-7

24. Bishop-Royse J. Quantitative systematic review of the index of concentration at the extremes. June 25, 2021. Unpublished.

25. Dougherty GB, Golden SH, Gross AL, Colantuoni E, Dean LT. Measuring structural racism and its association with BMI. *American Journal of Preventive Medicine*. 2020;59(4):530–537. doi:10.1016/j.amepre.2020.05.019

26. Graetz N, Esposito M. Historical redlining and contemporary racial disparities in neighborhood life expectancy. Published online October 20, 2021. doi:10.31235/osf.io/q9gbx

27. Houghton A, Jackson-Weaver O, Toraih E, et al. Firearm homicide mortality is influenced by structural racism in US metropolitan areas. *Journal of Trauma and Acute Care Surgery*. 2021;91(1):64–71. doi:10.1097/TA.0000000000003167

28. Krieger N, Van Wye G, Huynh M, et al. Structural racism, historical redlining, and risk of preterm birth in New York City, 2013–2017. *American Journal of Public Health*. 2020;110(7):1046–1053. doi:10.2105/AJPH.2020.305656

29. Larimore SH. *Routes to low birth weight (or not): Local, cultural racism in exceptional communities*. [PhD, University of Washington; 2019]. https://www.proquest.com/pqdtglobal/docview/2317596667/abstract/6523815FD2346F0PQ/2.

30. Liu SY, Fiorentini C, Bailey Z, Huynh M, McVeigh K, Kaplan D. Structural racism and severe maternal morbidity in New York State. *Clinical Medicine Insights. Women's Health.* 2019;12:1179562X19854778. doi:10.1177/1179562X19854778

31. Pabayo R, Ehntholt A, Davis K, Liu SY, Muennig P, Cook DM. Structural racism and odds for infant mortality among infants born in the United States 2010. *Journal of Racial and Ethnic Health Disparities.* 2019;6(6):1095–1106. doi:10.1007/s40615-019-00612-w

32. Siegel M, Critchfield-Jain I, Boykin M, Owens A. Actual racial/ethnic disparities in COVID-19 mortality for the non-Hispanic Black compared to non-Hispanic White population in 35 US States and their association with structural racism. *Journal of Racial and Ethnic Health Disparities.* Published online April 27, 2021. doi:10.1007/s40615-021-01028-1

33. Siegel M, Critchfield-Jain I, Boykin M, et al. Racial/ethnic disparities in state-level COVID-19 vaccination rates and their association with structural racism. *Journal of Racial and Ethnic Health Disparities.* Published online October 28, 2021. doi:10.1007/s40615-021-01173-7

34. Volpe VV, Schorpp KM, Cacace SC, Benson GP, Banos NC. State- and provider-level racism and health care in the U.S. *American Journal of Preventive Medicine.* 2021;61(3):338–347. doi:10.1016/j.amepre.2021.03.008

35. Owens-Young J, Bell CN. Structural racial inequities in socioeconomic status, urban-rural classification, and infant mortality in US counties. *Ethnicity & Disease.* 2020;30(3):389–398. doi:10.18865/ed.30.3.389

36. Shim RS. Dismantling structural racism in psychiatry: A path to mental health equity. *AJP.* 2021;178(7):592–598. doi:10.1176/appi.ajp.2021.21060558

37. Pohl DJ, Seblova D, Avila JF, et al. Relationship between residential segregation, later-life cognition, and incident dementia across race/ethnicity. *International Journal of Environmental Research and Public Health.* 2021;18(21). doi:10.3390/ijerph182111233

38. Mujahid MS, Gao X, Tabb LP, Morris C, Lewis TT. Historical redlining and cardiovascular health: The multi-ethnic study of atherosclerosis. *Proceedings of the National Academy of Sciences of the United States of America.* 2021;118(51). doi:10.1073/pnas.2110986118

39. Linton SL, Cooper HLF, Chen YT, et al. Mortgage discrimination and racial/ethnic concentration are associated with same-race/ethnicity partnering among people who inject drugs in 19 US Cities. *Journal of Urban Health.* 2020;97(1):88–104. doi:10.1007/s11524-019-00405-w

40. Leos C. *Examining the effect of state- and individual-level structural racism on Latino adolescent sexual risk behaviors: An intergroup and intragroup analysis.* [PhD, University of North Carolina, Chapel Hill; 2020]. *Dissertation Abstracts International Section A: Humanities and Social Sciences.* 2020;81(9-A).

41. Fernandez-Esquer ME, Ibekwe LN, Guerrero-Luera R, King YA, Durand CP, Atkinson JS. Structural racism and immigrant health: Exploring the association between wage theft, mental health, and injury among Latino day laborers. *Ethnicity & Disease.* 2021;31(Suppl 1):345–356. doi:10.18865/ed.31.S1.345

42. Butler B, Outrich M, Roach J, James A. Generational impacts of 1930s housing discrimination and the imperative need for the healthy start initiative to address structural racism. *Journal of Health Disparities Research and Practice.* 2020;13(3). https://digitalscholarship.unlv.edu/jhdrp/vol13/iss3/4

43. Chambers BD, Arabia SE, Arega HA, et al. Exposures to structural racism and racial discrimination among pregnant and early post-partum Black women living in Oakland, California. *Stress and Health.* 2020;36(2):213–219. doi:10.1002/smi.2922

44. Dyer L, Hardeman R, Vilda D, Theall K, Wallace M. Mass incarceration and public health: The association between black jail incarceration and adverse birth outcomes among black women in Louisiana. *BMC Pregnancy and Childbirth.* 2019;19(1):525. doi:10.1186/s12884-019-2690-z

45. Ibragimov U, Beane S, Friedman SR, et al. Police killings of Black people and rates of sexually transmitted infections: a cross-sectional analysis of 75 large US metropolitan

areas, 2016. *Sexually Transmitted Infections*. 2020;96(6):429–431. doi:10.1136/sextrans-2019-054026

46. Martz CD, Hunter EA, Kramer MR, et al. Pathways linking census tract typologies with subjective neighborhood disorder and depressive symptoms in the Black Women's Experiences Living with Lupus (BeWELL) Study. *Health & Place*. 2021;70:102587. doi:10.1016/j.healthplace.2021.102587

47. Richardson ET, Malik MM, Darity WA, et al. Reparations for Black American descendants of persons enslaved in the U.S. and their estimated impact on SARS-CoV-2 transmission. Published online June 5, 2020. doi:10.1101/2020.06.04.20112011

48. Tackett KJ, Jenkins F, Morrell DS, McShane DB, Burkhart CN. Structural racism and its influence on the severity of atopic dermatitis in African American children. *Pediatric Dermatology*. 2020;37(1):142–146. doi:10.1111/pde.14058

49. Bishop-Royse J, Lange-Maia B, Murray L, Shah RC, DeMaio F. Structural racism, socio-economic marginalization, and infant mortality. *Public Health*. 2021;190:55–61. doi:10.1016/j.puhe.2020.10.027

50. Brown J. *Structural factors and racial disparities in severe maternal morbidity: An examination of state-level indicators of structural racism and severe maternal morbidity among Black and White persons in the U.S., 2009–2011*. [Master's thesis. University of Washington; 2020]. https://www.proquest.com/pqdtglobal/docview/2493462764/abstract/6523815FD2346F0PQ/4.

51. Janevic T, Zeitlin J, Egorova NN, et al. Racial and economic neighborhood segregation, site of delivery, and morbidity and mortality in neonates born very preterm. *The Journal of Pediatrics*. 2021;235:116–123. doi:10.1016/j.jpeds.2021.03.049

52. Blebu BE, Ro A, Kane JB, Bruckner TA. An examination of preterm birth and residential social context among black immigrant women in California, 2007–2010. *Journal of Community Health*. 2019;44(5):857–865. doi:10.1007/s10900-018-00602-9

53. Samari G, Catalano R, Alcalá HE, Gemmill A. The Muslim Ban and preterm birth: Analysis of U.S. vital statistics data from 2009 to 2018. *Social Science & Medicine*. 2020;265:np. doi:10.1016/j.socscimed.2020.113544

54. Sudhinaraset M, Woofter R, Young Medt, Landrian A, Vilda D, Wallace SP. Analysis of state-level immigrant policies and preterm births by race/ethnicity among women born in the US and women born outside the US. *JAMA Network Open*. 2021;4(4):e214482. doi:10.1001/jamanetworkopen.2021.4482

55. Tan SB, deSouza P, Raifman M. Structural racism and COVID-19 in the USA: A county-level empirical analysis. *Journal of Racial and Ethnic Health Disparities*. 2021;9(1):236–246. doi:10.1007/s40615-020-00948-8

56. Mitchell J, Chihaya GK. Tract-level associations between historical residential redlining and contemporary fatal encounters with police. Published online October 7, 2021. doi:10.31235/osf.io/fu8rg

57. Islami F, Fedewa SA, Thomson B, Nogueira L, Yabroff KR, Jemal A. Association between disparities in intergenerational economic mobility and cause-specific mortality among Black and White persons in the United States. *Cancer Epidemiology*. 2021;74:101998. doi:10.1016/j.canep.2021.101998

58. Poulson M, Neufeld MY, Dechert T, Allee L, Kenzik KM. Historic redlining, structural racism, and firearm violence: A structural equation modeling approach. *The Lancet Regional Health—Americas*. 2021;3:100052. doi:10.1016/j.lana.2021.100052

59. Homan P, Brown TH, King B. Structural intersectionality as a new direction for health disparities research. *Journal of Health and Social Behavior*. 2021;62(3):350–370. doi:10.1177/00221465211032947

60. Fashaw-Walters SA, Rahman M, Gee G, Mor V, White M, Thomas KS. Out of reach: Inequities in the use of high-quality home health agencies. *Health Affairs*. 2022;41(2):247–255. doi:10.1377/hlthaff.2021.01408

61. Kramer MR, Hogue CR. Is segregation bad for your health? *Epidemiologic Reviews*. 2009;31(1):178–194. doi:10.1093/epirev/mxp001

62. Williams DR, Collins C. Racial residential segregation: A fundamental cause of racial disparities in health. *Public Health Reports.* 2001;116:13.

63. Treuhaft S, Langston A, Scoggins J, Lee J, Pastor M. The Racial Equity Index: A new data tool to drive local efforts to dismantle structural racism. *National Equity Atlas.* July 23, 2020. https://nationalequityatlas.org/research/index-findings.

64. Krieger N. Methods for the scientific study of discrimination and health: An ecosocial approach. *American Journal of Public Health.* 2012;102(5):936–944. doi:10.2105/AJPH.2011.300544

65. Geronimus AT. The weathering hypothesis and the health of African-American women and infants: Evidence and speculations. *Ethnicity & Disease.* 1992;2(3):207–221.

66. Riley AR. *The social production of health inequalities across state and regional contexts.* Chicago: University of Chicago Press; 2019. doi:10.6082/uchicago.1856

67. Chantarat T, Mentzer KM, Van Riper DC, Hardeman RR. Where are the labor markets?: Examining the association between structural racism in labor markets and infant birth weight. *Health & Place.* 2022;74:102742. doi:10.1016/j.healthplace.2022.102742

68. Acharya A, Blackwell M, Sen M. A culture of disenfranchisement: How American slavery continues to affect voting behavior. 2015. https://mattblackwell.org/research/slavery-voting/.

69. Hing A. *Suppressing the vote, suppressing future voters: A multilevel analysis of voter suppression and Black–White disparities in life expectancy and infant outcomes.* [PhD, UCLA; 2021]. https://escholarship.org/uc/item/6q03q08t.

70. Kirk MA, Kelley C, Yankey N, Birken SA, Abadie B, Damschroder L. A systematic review of the use of the Consolidated Framework for Implementation Research. *Implementation Science.* 2016;11(1):72. doi:10.1186/s13012-016-0437-z

71. Hernan MA. Estimating causal effects from epidemiological data. *Journal of Epidemiology & Community Health.* 2006;60(7):578–586. doi:10.1136/jech.2004.029496

72. Pearl J. Causal inference in statistics: An overview. *Statistics Survey.* 2009;3:np. doi:10.1214/09-SS057

73. Robins J. A graphical approach to the identification and estimation of causal parameters in mortality studies with sustained exposure periods. *Journal of Chronic Diseases.* 1987;40:139S–161S. doi:10.1016/S0021-9681(87)80018-8

74. Lett E, Adekunle D, McMurray P, et al. Health equity tourism: Ravaging the justice landscape. *Journal of Medical Systems.* 2022;46(3):17. doi:10.1007/s10916-022-01803-5

75. Gee GC, Walsemann KM, Brondolo E. A life course perspective on how racism may be related to health inequities. *American Journal of Public Health.* 2012;102(5):967–974. doi:10.2105/AJPH.2012.300666

76. Gee GC, Hing A, Mohammed S, Tabor DC, Williams DR. Racism and the life course: Taking time seriously. *American Journal of Public Health.* 2019;109(S1):S43–S47. doi:10.2105/AJPH.2018.304766

77. Kang-Brown J. Incarceration trends. *Vera Institute of Justice*; 2022. https://www.vera.org/projects/incarceration-trends.

78. Bertoni N, Keeter S. How to access Pew Research Center survey data. *Pew Research Center*; October 22, 2021. https://www.pewresearch.org/fact-tank/2021/10/22/how-to-access-pew-research-center-survey-data/.

79. GHDx. Global burden of disease collaborative network. Published 2022. https://ghdx.healthdata.org/organizations/global-burden-disease-collaborative-network.

80. Eviction Lab. *Eviction map & data.* Accessed April 29, 2022. https://evictionlab.org/map/.

81. National Conference of State Legislatures. Legislative news, studies and analysis. Accessed April 29, 2022. https://www.ncsl.org/.

82. The Stanford Open Policing Project. Data. Accessed April 29, 2022. https://openpolicing.stanford.edu/.

5

Lessons from the Urban Institute's Demonstration Projects

Chitra Balakrishnan, Rekha Balu, Claire Cusella,
and Karishma Furtado

Introduction

Despite a long-standing and growing body of research showing how structural racism operates, many issue experts continue to study race as an individual characteristic rather than to analyze how racism permeates social, political, and economic processes. At the same time, those at the cutting edge of structural racism research often focus more on exposing injustices than equipping policymakers with actionable recommendations in the context of specific policy debates. As a result, there is relatively little policy research grounded in structural analysis that also presents policy solutions. The field requires new methods and approaches for policy-oriented social science research.

To address this need, in 2021 the Robert Wood Johnson Foundation (RWJF) awarded the Urban Institute a grant for a demonstration project called "Interrupting Structural Racism's Impact on Health and Wellbeing." Over thirteen months, this project supported five demonstration studies conducted by Urban Institute research teams in consultation with experts in equity-focused research and analysis. Each study sought to analyze the role of structural racism as a causal driver of outcomes in a particular policy area to increase understanding of why racial disparities persist and how systemic changes could produce more equitable outcomes. Urban's new Office of Race and Equity Research managed the portfolio of projects, and provided the demonstration teams with literature, conceptual as well as technical review, resource materials, coaching and extensive feedback at critical stages of the research process.

Chitra Balakrishnan, Rekha Balu, Claire Cusella, and Karishma Furtado, *Lessons from the Urban Institute's Demonstration Projects*. In: *Research to Action*. Edited by: Claire Gibbons and Alonzo L. Plough, Oxford University Press. © Robert Wood Johnson Foundation (2026). DOI: 10.1093/9780197819876.003.0006

We did not expect that a year-long project of this kind would be sufficient to produce fully realized examples of transformative research or innovative new methods of structural policy analysis. Yet we were surprised and humbled by how challenging it was to help colleagues incorporate more historical, multi-level and multi-systems perspectives—from the way studies are designed and implemented to their findings and recommendations—even when teams were highly motivated to do so. To a greater degree than we expected, researchers need an extensive array of supports to challenge disciplinary and field norms that can obscure structural racism, norms that insist on isolating causes *within* rather than *across* systems, and that undervalue historical analysis. There is also a need for more creative approaches to fostering collaboration, so that those most fluent in structural racism analysis (be they early or later in their career) lead these studies.

The project affirmed three key lessons. First, it showed that change *is* possible, and that teams learn by doing. Each of the studies surfaced insights that would not have been possible without structural analysis, and many of the researchers involved made progress in their willingness and capacity to identify structural racism as a driver of racial disparity. They have demonstrated this increased capacity in subsequent work.

Second, efforts to transform the way we work need more *time*: time for researchers to continually interrogate their assumptions, to read and reflect on foundational texts, to build trust with community members and practitioners who bring critical insights, and to experiment to overcome challenges. The project's short timeline resulted from aspirations to inform strategy development processes then underway at both Urban and RWJF. Efforts to confront structural racism are often inhibited by this kind of time pressure, which is endemic to policy research. Research organizations and funders can help transform the field by taking a longer and more realistic view of the work required to fulfill equity commitments.

Third, isolated efforts to build capacity are insufficient to create *institutional* change, which is necessary if policy research is to play a much more significant role in disrupting structural racism. The Urban Institute has adopted and supported a comprehensive Race and Equity Framework to advance this kind of institutional change. Our Office of Race and Equity Research grew out of this framework and will apply the lessons from this demonstration project iteratively in the years ahead. Success will depend on collaborating with many researchers from different disciplines across many projects. Success will also depend on efforts outside of individual research projects to change organizational culture and disrupt structural racism within Urban and the broader policy research field.

This chapter describes the demonstration projects, shares our lessons in more detail, and offers recommendations for funders and researchers who share our goals.

Our Approach

We set up a project where research teams learn by doing—by moving from the stages of proposal development to project design to analysis and interpretation. This is how research teams typically acquire their expertise, and how we think research teams can also develop fluency in structural racism research. Assembling teams of experienced and new researchers, those who can bring topical and research methods experience and those who can bring a historical and ecological framework to understanding systems of privilege and exclusion, also sets the stage for learning. We aim to cultivate not only new projects, but also new kinds of research questions and new types of inquiry. We recognized that one project would not be sufficient to shift years of training, but saw this as a starting place for new inquiry.

The emerging, interdisciplinary field of structural racism research will gain momentum and attract new scholarship by reflecting on what study teams find easy or difficult. This chapter shares our learnings from an attempt to translate our commitment to racial equity into action within our specific culture as a research organization. Interest in understanding and dismantling structural racism is growing across the policy research field. While this is promising, the field is still at a relatively early stage of development. Research teams still require more time and financial support to absorb and apply the relevant literature than they do when conducting more traditional research.

Project Description

Selection and Staffing of the Demonstration Studies

This effort to demonstrate approaches to addressing structural racism in policy research was conceived in part to inform strategy development processes then underway at both Urban and RWJF. To serve this purpose, the demonstration studies had to be completed within a compressed time frame, which resulted in an expedited process for identifying the five demonstration studies. We issued an informal call for ideas to researchers across Urban and generated nearly 40 brief submissions from colleagues working in many different issue areas. We developed a scoring rubric and invited finalists to develop their ideas further in consultation with the leadership team. This resulted in the five studies described in this chapter, which were published in late 2022 and early 2023.

During the selection process, we asked our colleagues to conceptualize structural racism in two ways for this project. First, we drew on Urban's definition from an internal toolkit on structural racism:

> Structural racism is the feature of our social, economic, and political systems in which an array of dynamics—historical, institutional, cultural, and interpersonal—legitimize and reinforce racial inequity. These dynamics facilitate and maintain advantages for White people while creating and maintaining disadvantage and barriers to opportunity and well-being for people of color. Structural racism creates disparities in access to opportunity, ability to take advantage of opportunities, and the likelihood that taking advantage of opportunities will yield equitable outcomes . . . the disparities it creates often persist or compound across generations.

Second, we asked that the teams consider structural racism primarily a *cause*, a mediator, and/or a set of contextual factors that resides at the level of systems and policies. Causal or contextual analysis often requires historical analysis, specifically attention to an evolution and accumulation of policy and cultural actions that create and sustain systems of disadvantage. This analysis is distinct from analysis of racial inequity, which is an *outcome*, or product, of structural racism. Therefore, a focus on structural racism requires moving upstream from racial inequity to better understand underlying drivers and causes (including policies) in order to conduct research and design policies that do not just treat the "symptoms" of racial inequality but work toward prevention and "cures."

Each of the demonstration teams brought deep expertise in their issue areas, a track record of success in conducting influential policy research, and motivation to help expose and remedy racial inequities. They had varying, and generally limited, familiarity with structural racism literature, and they reflected the demographic makeup of Urban's research staff:

senior researchers, who are predominantly White, working with increasingly diverse early- and mid-career colleagues. The study teams included experts who had never before named or described structural racism in their published work and who have gone on to do so in other projects.

Supports for the Demonstration Studies

In order to support the participating researchers, we assembled a primarily BIPOC leadership and advisory team that brought extensive experience studying racial inequality in policy and practice across issue areas. This group included the founding co-Vice President of Urban's Office of Race and Equity Research (ORER), which launched in 2022; several experts who came to Urban through our equity scholars program[1]; and several colleagues and an external expert with relevant subject matter expertise.

This team offered ongoing and episodic supports to the researchers conducting the demonstration studies. We held monthly check-ins with each team, offering feedback on every step of the process: research questions, protocols, literature reviews, outlines, and drafts. Advisors offered early feedback on initial outlines and wrote a reflection memo after reviewing the first draft.

During our regular check-in and feedback meetings, we also talked with teams about various purposes of structural racism research and how they could operationalize one or more of those in their project, including these examples:

- **Increasing awareness**: Naming and identifying systems, documenting examples of where and how structural racism manifests, and with what effects. This often involves descriptive research, drawing on a wide range of quantitative and qualitative data, including observations, maps, interviews.[2]
- **Identifying persistent system-level barriers and constraints**: May involve historical analysis to show persistence of barriers and systems of exclusion over time, and may require different data collection or analyses than typical individual-level analyses.

---

[1] https://www.urban.org/urban-institute-equity-scholars.
[2] See Hobson JM, Moody MD, Sorge RE, Goodin BR. The neurobiology of social stress resulting from racism: Implications for pain disparities among racialized minorities. *Neurobiology of Pain.* 2022;12: 100101.

- **Measuring structural racism in new ways, or ways that build on existing evidence**: The measurement of structural racism is still under debate. Researchers within and between disciplines are asking questions such as whether we measure structural racism as a cause at the community or individual level (or both); measure it at a point in time or over an extended period; measure it as extreme concentration of (in)opportunity, or as disproportionate burden; or consider it as policies that actively restrict access or use of resources.[3] Each of these approaches may require different types of data and methodological approaches, and all may be necessary to include.
- **Evaluating the effectiveness of new structural interventions**: The researcher may look at structural racism as having a single and/or observable causal pathway that can be modified with a new intervention. One can then follow more typical program evaluation frameworks.
- **Designing proposals for future policy and practice change**: Solve for how structural racism persists across, and because of, the mutually reinforcing and interlocking nature of systems.[4]

We also shared internally developed resources like Urban's Structural Racism Explainer Collection,[5] and reflection and guidance documents.[6]

To help the demonstration study teams with writing, the advisory team asked before they started their first draft how their research would provide new evidence on structural racism and drivers of disparities, what they are learning about potential mechanisms to interrupt structural racism, and what approaches or frames they are using for their results and policy recommendations. After the outline and first draft, internal and external reviewers provided detailed feedback on opportunities to reframe and incorporate a structural racism analysis.

---

[3] See Lorraine T. Dean and Roland J. Thorpe, Jr. 2022. "What Structural Racism Is (or Is Not) and How to Measure It: Clarity for Public Health and Medical Researchers." *American Journal of Epidemiology* 191 (9): 1521–1526; Paris B. Adkins-Jackson, Tongtan Chantarat, Zinzi D. Bailey, and Ninez A. Ponce. 2022. "Measuring Structural Racism: A Guide for Epidemiologists and Other Health Researchers." American Journal of Epidemiology 191 (4): 539–547.

[4] As an example, RWJF's climate change series seeks to propose solutions that address the challenges of multiple systems. "Climate Change Threatens our Health and Deepens Health Inequities." Robert Wood Johnson Foundation, September 2021. https://www.rwjf.org/en/library/research/2021/09/climate-change-threatens-our-health-and-deepens-health-inequities.html.

[5] Margery A. Turner, Solomon Greene, Tomás Monarrez, Martha Galvez, Peace Gwam, and Mychal Cohen, n.d., "Structural Racism Explainer Collection," Urban Institute, https://www.urban.org/projects/structural-racism-explainer-collection.

[6] See Steven Brown, Kilolo Kijakazi, Charmaine Runes, and Margery A. Turner. 2019. "Confronting Structural Racism in Research and Policy Analysis." Washington, DC: Urban Institute.

The Projects

The five completed demonstration studies, each studying a distinct policy area, pursued questions of different scope and were each rich in their own way. Below is a high-level summary of the primary research question, methods used, findings and policy recommendations.

Transportation Policy—Disrupting Structural Racism: Increasing Transportation Equity in South Dallas

In response to a request from a South Dallas-based transportation group, this project sought to identify structural solutions to transportation inequities in South Dallas and other regions, drawing on local interviews as well as a community-engaged feasibility analysis. To better understand the needs of the residents and their transportation-related barriers to economic opportunity, the team interviewed local stakeholders in South Dallas, analyzing historical drivers and interlocking systems that contributed to racial and other disparities in service availability, infrastructure, and resources using interview data and synthesizing existing research. They also conducted case studies of four other parts of the country with similar challenges (identified with quantitative analysis). The team found that intentional equity improvements, such as increased transportation access for low-wage workers, resulted from wide-reaching changes to transportation decision-making processes rather than from particular individual policies and programs. They recommended that local leaders make these changes through mechanisms such as equity councils, and that they prioritize deep community engagement early on to build solutions in partnership with community members. They also encouraged a cross-sector approach to transportation equity via collaboration with land use, community development, and housing entities.

Behavioral Health Policy—Disrupting Structural Racism's Impact on Health and Well-Being for People Who Use Substances: Recommendations for Programs and Funders from Key Informant Interviews

This project sought to determine how previous studies, assessments, and tools identified and characterized services in the community that address structural racism. The study also explored the needs of people who use substances, as well as how local organizations and programs can provide services that counter structural racism with respect to substance use. The team conducted an environmental scan of studies, identified assets and services in communities that address the needs of people who use substances, and conducted nine interviews with practitioner leaders involved in community-based programs and organizations that provide culturally and linguistically responsive substance use services. They recommended that funders support the use of participant (client) boards to identify culturally effective care and services. They also recommended that funders adopt a greater role in supporting racial justice work by supporting smaller service providers that offer intentionally non-punitive and anti-racist services for substance users, as well as by involving the community in grantmaking and prioritizing grantees' community-based research agendas. Their policy recommendation is to build new structures and systems that redistribute resources from structurally racist systems, such as the criminal-legal system.

Child Welfare Policy—Prevention Services Availability and Black–White Placement Disparity: Contextualizing Structural Racism in Child Welfare
This project aimed to identify whether differences in the availability of child welfare prevention services were related to racial disparities in foster care placement rates. This project analyzed whether the structures, functions, and capacities of county child welfare systems differ between areas where the differences in the proportion of Black children placed in foster care versus White children is smaller compared with areas where it is larger. The study team conducted an environmental scan, site observation, and semi-structured interviews with service administrators. The study found preliminary evidence for and against their hypothesis that areas of high White economic disadvantage would have more placement services than areas of similar Black economic disadvantage. The study offered a few hypotheses for the finding that areas with higher White child placement rates had fewer prevention services. Ideas included perceptions of Black families' risk and need as potentially higher, White resistance to the location of prevention services in their communities, and delayed resource allocation to match the geographic distribution of placements. The paper concludes that further research is needed, including further examination of differential preventive services allocation and perceptions of those services as alternatives to placement, more in-depth ethnographic methods with observations and interviews with a broad range of community members and stakeholders, and analysis of administrative data to determine whether racial disparity exists in both voluntary and court-mandated referrals. Such analysis could be particularly useful as jurisdictions seek to reduce and prevent unnecessary child placement in foster care under the federal Families First Prevention Services Act.

Tax Policy—Racial Disparities in the Income Tax Treatment of Marriage
This project aimed to determine whether, and to what extent, the federal individual income tax results in racial disparities (via marriage penalties and bonuses) between Black married couples and White married couples. The team converted household data from the Survey of Consumer Finances into tax units and input this information into the TAXSIM model to calculate tax liabilities. The research found that under 2018 tax law, Black couples in all income brackets faced larger and more frequent penalties compared to their White counterparts. The authors noted that the tax code relies on several economic inputs that reflect structural racism, such as overall income, whether spouses earn comparable or different amounts, and family structure and size (the number of dependents); as a result, these factors can produce racial disparities in tax liabilities. Comparing marriage penalties in 2000, 2015, and 2018, they also found that Black married couples were more likely than White married couples to face penalties in all years, with disparities increasing over time. The authors assessed the effects of two policy changes (allowing spouses to choose to file jointly or singly, and reinstating the two-earner deduction) on Black and White earners. The team recommended that policymakers consider the implications for racial equity and potential differential impacts of future changes to the tax treatment of marriage.

Retirement Policy—How Structural Racism and Limits on Economic Opportunity Restrict Social Security Benefits for Black Retirees
This project sought to quantify how reducing or eliminating racial disparities in key life outcomes influences Social Security payouts. Using the Urban Institute's dynamic microsimulation model, DYNASIM4, the team simulated Social Security benefits for Black and White workers nearing retirement (born in 1996 to 2005) based on historically observed racial differences in educational attainment, wages, employment, mortality, disability and health problems, and marital history. The study estimated that annual Social Security payments for Black beneficiaries at age 70 are 25 percent lower and average lifetime payments are 18 percent lower compared to their White counterparts. The team then forecasted how much benefits for Black retirees would increase if those racial disparities were no longer present. The study confirmed that the systemic disadvantages in education, employment and health faced by Black workers while working reduce their annual and lifetime Social Security benefits upon retirement. The authors found that although Social Security was designed to be progressive by age, some features of the program do not account for other intersectional needs

for progressivity, namely not adjusting for higher rates of mortality among Black households compared to White and not compensating single heads of household and working-class households for a lifetime of lower earnings and wealth.

In sum, each project found racial dimensions in the implementation of each of the policies studied, something that would not have been discovered without at least an equity analysis. They also illustrate the benefit of pairing subject matter experts who know the inner workings of a policy system with a structural framework.

To be sure, each project could have dug deeper. Although each project had a different external reviewer, comments across projects tended to focus on similar themes, and called for:

- Deeper engagement review of relevant scholarship on racial equity and structural racism;
- More discussion of other systems at play (e.g., relationship between housing, jobs and income, rather than just talking about income as if it were independent);
- More weight to be given to structural racism or racial disparities than other policy challenges, precisely because of the interdependence between systems; and acknowledgement that policy solutions that would address these racist structures are necessarily, rather than excessively, complicated;
- Analytic changes to avoid calling a racial characteristic a measure of racism, and to meet the need for other variables, models and methods to get at the effects of racism;
- Interviews with those directly affected by the policy being studied, and for voices and experiences in addition to quantitative estimates;
- Stronger policy solutions, rather than incremental and/or programmatic changes that can be reversed easily.

Reflections from Project Teams

Overall, the five study teams appreciated the opportunity to participate in a project focused on structural racism but found the timeline too short and frustrating. In addition, there was some confusion about whose direction to follow—RWJF as the funder, the external reviewer as the subject expert, or ORER as the project manager.

Teams stressed the value of the external reviewers in providing substantive comments on the paper. One team noted that the connection to their external reviewer has also allowed them to participate in other opportunities with researchers engaged in structural racism research.

Teams also reflected on the timing of feedback. One team found that early discussions with the ORER team played the greatest role in shaping their project. However, another team observed that the scholars and external reviewers could have helped more if they had been on board and involved earlier in the project, before data collection began. The feedback still informed later rounds of the team's data collection, but the project's quick timeline made it difficult to make as many adjustments as they would have liked.

Study teams found the resources shared by the ORER team helpful (see Box 5.1). Two study leads acknowledged that this project marked the first time they made structural racism the primary focus of their research. One noted that it offered the opportunity to clarify the difference between structural and nonstructural solutions. They expressed that the iterative nature of the project, in working alongside the ORER team and the external reviewers, allowed them to consider each step in the research process through a structural lens.

Box 5.1 Examples of Guidance and Resources Shared with Project Teams

---

Throughout the project, we shared resources with the project leads to build on their understanding of structural racism.

- Systemic and Structural Racism: Definitions, Examples, Health Damages, and Approaches to Dismantling[7]
- How the Effects of Racial Bias Compound[8]
- The Economic Cost of Racial Inequality[9]
- Changing Power Dynamics among Researchers, Local Governments, and Community Members[10]
- National Academies Panel on Structural Racism[11]
- Structural Racism and Rigorous Models of Social Inequity: Proceedings of a Workshop (2022)[12]
- Rethinking Racism: Towards a Structural Interpretation[13]

continued

continued

- Urban internal resources:
  – Structural Racism Resource Library
  – Applying a Structural Racism Lens to Research Toolkit

[7] Paula A. Braveman, Elaine Arkin, Dwayne Proctor, Tina Kauh, and Nicole Holm. 2022. "Systemic and Structural Racism: Definitions, Examples, Health Damages, and Approaches to Dismantling." *Health Affairs* 41 (2): 171–178.

[8] "How the Effects of Racial Bias Compound," RAND Corporation, accessed December 27, 2022, https://www.rand.org/pubs/tools/TLA960-1/tool.html.

[9] Kate Davidson and Aubree E. Weaver, "The Economic Cost of Racial Inequality," July 21, 2022, https://www.politico.com/newsletters/morning-money/2022/07/21/the-economic-cost-of-racial-inequality-00047025.

[10] Sonia Torres Rodríguez, Mikaela Tajo, Shamoiya Washington, and Kimberly Burrowes. 2022. *Changing Power Dynamics among Researchers, Local Governments, and Community Members.* Washington, DC: Urban Institute.

[11] "Structural Racism and Rigorous Models of Social Inequity: A Workshop," National Academies of Sciences, Engineering and Medicine, May 16–17, 2022, https://www.nationalacademies.org/event/05-16-2022/structural-racism-and-rigorous-models-of-social-inequity-a-workshop.

[12] National Academies of Sciences, Engineering, and Medicine. 2022. *Structural Racism and Rigorous Models of Social Inequity: Proceedings of a Workshop. Washington, DC: The National Academies Press.*

[13] Eduardo Bonilla-Silva. 1994. "Rethinking Racism: Towards a Structural Interpretation." Center for Research on Social Organization Working Paper 526. Ann Arbor: University of Michigan.

Reflections from External and Internal Reviewers

Both internal and external reviewers noted that this project represented both a challenge and an opportunity as the researchers possessed such differing levels of exposure and experience with structural racism. They agreed with demonstration study teams that earlier involvement of race and equity scholars could have improved the research process and strengthened early drafts. Reviewers emphasized how collaboration has been so key to their work in structural racism and observed it as a crucial step in improving these demonstration studies; the silos that have been created in academic studies are not reflective of how oppression operates, and working with colleagues across disciplines can significantly strengthen the research process and contextual findings within other systems that are contributing to disparities. As an example, the reviewer of the child welfare report encouraged the researchers to consider and discuss racialized poverty as it relates to child protective services exposure and involvement. The Social Security team was encouraged to consider labor force participation more broadly and how healthcare and housing discrimination could have downstream effects on retirees' benefits.

In reviewing first drafts, nearly all of the internal and external reviewers noted that the papers needed to engage more with recent scholarship on racial equity and structural racism to contextualize their research questions, analysis, and recommendations. One reviewer captured the essence of several reviewers' comments when they noted that part of applying an anti-oppressive approach with a social justice lens to such research inquiries requires mindfulness of the literature typically propped up as the gold standard of empirical evidence. It's important to remain cognizant of the race and ethnicity, and social positions of the scholars typically cited for reporting on marginalized people of color, whilst other scholarship from members of those communities gets short shrift. To dismantle structural biases at all steps of our scholarly processes, we need to be reflective of inherent hierarchies regarding who is privileged to conduct and disseminate the research.

Reviewers encouraged researchers to reflect on their own positionalities and research team makeups and to make that explicit in their reports given the nature of the inquiries regarding race. Reviewers emphasized the need for community engagement and perspectives from those with lived experience in both the research team and in the data collection.

Several of the reviewers, both internally and externally, reflected on the difficulties in serving in an advisory role such as this. It felt taxing and burdensome for some reviewers to introduce the funded study teams to structural racism as a lived experience and a whole area of research in such a short amount of time. One reviewer noted that "[traditional] studies are suited to document disparities, they are less useful in explaining why they exist" and thus researchers have to innovate in their methods to get at the effects of racism. Occasional hesitancy from some researchers to adjust their approach, particularly when the suggested approach includes considering literature and methods outside of one's disciplinary training, engaging stakeholders in new ways, and so on also felt challenging. Some reviewers also noted that this is why advising is not sufficient; co-authorship between issue experts and race and equity experts would be a better approach to ensure that structural racism is taken seriously and incorporated throughout.

We are grateful to our external reviewers (Dorothy Brown, Mikki Waid, Matthew Freedman, Tracie Gardner, and Darcey Merritt) and internal reviewers (Brian Smedley, Karishma Furtado, Michael Neal, Luisa Godinez-Puig, and Shauna Cooper) for their contributions to the demonstration studies and the project as a whole.

Key Challenges Related to Embedding a Structural Racism Lens

We observed some common sticking points and implicit needs for researchers across these projects. These were just five studies in a single institution—while our sample is small and not randomly selected, the studies reflect common team compositions and experience levels and the challenges reflected in other literature on data equity and critical perspectives on race. The project focused on a set of researchers who were likely in the middle of the distribution when it comes to interest in, awareness of, and readiness for implementing a structural racism lens in their research. Focusing on the middle could be a different way to embed new approaches and practices by shifting and advancing the average practice. It also takes more work on the part of the teams and the advisers.

To truly embed structural racism would involve researchers adopting new ways of working, not just participating in a one-off or new research project. In this section, we outline some of the challenges to spur those new ways of working, which then set up our final section of recommendations to funders.

1) Privileging Seniority and Credentials Reinforces Hierarchies, Precisely What a Structural Racism Lens Is Meant to Shift

The demonstration project teams included researchers with nearly 40 years of experience as well as newly graduated research assistants. However, in nearly all of our advising meetings and email exchanges, only the principal investigators (PIs) or co-PIs were present or responding, which may have inhibited our advice from being more deeply integrated across the project. This design meant that we were reliant on the senior researchers to accept and communicate our team's or reviewer's suggestions on their approach. Early-career researchers who have recently graduated from doctoral training may have more relevant experience, training, and familiarity with the frameworks and definitions for analyzing structural racism than those who are more senior or distant from this new research frontier. Therefore, a shared leadership model could bring together multiple kinds of expertise in a more collaborative format than the traditional top-down format. The field should not ignore new voices any more than it should disregard the knowledge that comes with seniority.

2) Systems-level Analysis Requires a Different Analytic Framework for Both Quantitative and Qualitative Researchers

While social science and public health researchers have been trained and bring experience in noting disparities by race, many are less experienced at moving beyond these disparities to investigate root causes.

The research teams in this project took different analytical stances on whether structural racism was a cause, an effect, and/or a contextual factor; and used different methodologies (e.g., interviews, administrative data analysis, mixed methods, simulations). All used empirical approaches that they were familiar with and focused on data in their current study (rather than an accumulation of studies across disciplines), which could have limited the willingness to name something as structural. (We note that most projects analyzed structural racism primarily against Black communities, rather than all race and ethnic groups). Most of the analysis was correlational (although project teams initially conceptualized their work as causal) and focused on point-in-time differences in outcomes between Black and White households or communities (rather than an analysis of how structures cumulatively create disadvantage). These point-in-time comparisons may have been related to a tendency to minimize historical factors that have contributed to and compounded structural disadvantages.

The project timeline did not allow for application of new methodologies emerging from public health or other disciplines to analyze intersectional or compounding effects, for example.[14] Even the tax policy and retirement

[14] For example, see Clare R. Evans, David R. Williams, Jukka-Pekka Onnela, and S. V. Subramanian. 2018. "A Multilevel Approach to Modeling Health Inequalities at the Intersection of Multiple Social Identities." *Social Science & Medicine* 203 (2018): 64–73; Nick Graetz, Courtney E. Boen, and Michael H. Esposito. 2022 "Structural Racism and Quantitative Causal Inference: A Life Course Mediation Framework for Decomposing Racial Health Disparities." *Journal of Health and Social Behavior* 63 (2): 232–249; and Geoff B. Dougherty, Sherita H. Golden, Alden L. Gross, Elizabeth

policy projects' simulation analyses, which are relatively new to social sciences themselves, set up their models to forecast an estimated average effect, and then between-group differences in that average effect, rather than modeling heterogeneity itself as the pattern of interest.[15]

This approach to analysis also reflects, in part, that default quantitative analytic frameworks are set up to model race as an individual characteristic rather than racism as a multiple systems-level characteristic that would therefore have ripple effects on virtually every other variable at multiple levels (individual, community, administrative, etc.). In addition, more common analytic frameworks are not well set up to address intersectional effects (which require modeling multi-level and cross-classified phenomena). Qualitative frameworks also were limited by initial definitions that teams used, the way questions were phrased, and the underlying premise those reflected about how structural racism (rather than interpersonal racism) operates. Interviewees, whether of the same or different races as interviewers, are uncomfortable discussing structural racism in response to direct questions, and need other approaches to disclose or describe experiences in ways that reveal implicit structures.

3) Structural Analysis Sits Outside of any Single Disciplinary Training or System

Researchers are trained to address a narrow research question with a specific method. The inherent tension between researchers' need to address a well-defined research question and zooming out to the more global framework was present throughout the project. For example, we encouraged the transportation and tax policy teams to expand on their findings and explain how other sectors influenced the one they studied—for example, the role of historical zoning and limits on land use in Dallas were tools to isolate communities of color and therefore examples of structural racism's mechanisms.

Colantuoni, and Lorraine T. Dean. 2020. "Measuring Structural Racism and Its Association With BMI." *American Journal of Preventative Medicine* 59 (4): 530–537. https://pubmed.ncbi.nlm.nih.gov/29199054/.

  [15] Miratrix, L. W., Weiss, M. J., and Henderson, B. 2021. "An Applied Researcher's Guide to Estimating Effects from Multisite Individually Randomized Trials: Estimands, Estimators, and Estimates." *Journal of Research on Educational Effectiveness* 14 (1): 270–308. https://doi.org/10.1080/19345747.2020.1831115.

Further, researchers' specific disciplinary training and subject matter expertise seemed to collide with the proposition that structural racism analysis must contend with features of multiple reinforcing systems. Initially, most research teams said they felt like we were asking them to extrapolate beyond their expertise and knowledge, and perhaps even beyond what the data and analysis showed. This may reflect a focus on the current point in time, or a lack of consideration of analysis accumulated over decades. This poses a notable challenge when attempting to study structural racism, which has been built upon and exacerbated by decades of past policies and practices. Researchers' lack of experience with structural racism literature limited their comfort with discussing history and making claims or inferences from multiple disciplines, compared with claims they felt comfortable making relative to their own discipline. This narrow focus can have the unintended effect of minimizing discussion of the impacts of structural racism.

Even among researchers who want to address the role of multiple systems, the face disciplinary and subject matter norms—enforced by journal editors, conferences, and other gatekeeping entities—that insist on isolating causes within rather than across systems. These barriers are reinforced over years and cannot be unlearned in one project.

4) Researchers Need to See Structural Racism as a System of Systems, and Make Inferences Accordingly

We expected that teams would turn to the theories and literature on structural racism we shared (see Box 5.1 for examples) to inform their decisions about analysis and analytical approach. Some teams already had a stable of references, some referred to the provided resources, while others did not cite them at all in the initial drafts. Second drafts improved as teams addressed reviewer comments, incorporated reviewer-suggested references, and updated discussions. For other teams, when discussion of structural racism did appear, it appeared as an add-on paragraph, rather than being integrated throughout the paper. Notably, feedback came too late in the project life cycle for teams to change the analytic approach in ways that would allow them to infer or make conclusions related to structural racism based on their data collection.

When providing feedback, reviewers (including some of the authors of this chapter) encouraged teams to consider why and how we would expect different policies to operate in ways that reflect and reinforce structural racism—and why looking for this connection is not groundless speculation but rather opening up new areas and types of inquiry about interdependent systems (which call for new measurement, methodological or conceptual approaches). Some teams incorporated this feedback as they considered policy recommendations and areas for future research. Other teams struggled with making inferences beyond their narrow research question and specific dataset, even if literature in adjacent policy areas had documented structural racism via housing segregation, educational inequality, and other relevant phenomena.

Organizational Change Strategies Required

Researchers' comfort or willingness to consider new methods, anchor in existing and emerging theory, and imagine and recommend structural interventions are, of course, not just about them as individuals—they reflect the structures that encourage those patterns and the norms and models that sustain those structures. One relevant default structure at Urban is the convention of appointing the most senior person on a project to be its leader. Another is a standard project lifecycle that is too short and that rushes through the entire research process, including particularly important aspects relevant for structural racism work including foundation setting (e.g., naming assumptions, grounding in theory, and determining approach). A third is inviting feedback from a limited cast of characters (usually other researchers) in a hurried and superficial way, oftentimes later in the project (e.g., when writing up findings), when it is too late for teams to make substantial changes in response to recommendations about the fundamental research question and approach.

Urban did not forge these structures in a vacuum. On one side, funders often look for conventional measures of success (e.g., seniority, length of publication record) or lean on their long-standing relationships with researchers, all of which prize tenure. Funders, via funding priorities and parameters for a given opportunity, also set the frame within which researchers issue their proposals. In addition, patterns of funding and targeting resources are themselves a legacy of racism and eurocentrism, with efficiency-based metrics currently used to determine project leadership (number of years of experience, number of articles produced, relatively short timeframes for impact). On the other side, project leaders then tend to be the individuals who received the funding for the project based on tenure-related measures of skill and propose a research project scope that fits within funding and time constraints.

Ultimately, we need to shift from incremental change strategies in occasional projects to transforming the way we conceptualize research questions and approaches. These structures, built and reinforced by Urban, the field of research, and the widening concentric circles that surround and support it, also emanate from a set of mental models that we must name and reform if we want to achieve enduring change. For instance, in research (and arguably well beyond), we tend to believe that the scientific process is the best way of producing knowledge. As a result, we assume scientists know best, that scientists with more experience doing science know better than scientists with less experience, that quantitative data are more valid than qualitative, and that we grow the edifice of knowledge brick-by-brick, which is to say incrementally, through research that asks similarly incremental questions. Even broader societal values of prizing outcomes (the end point) over outputs (the process) were also at work. These are just some of the mental models that are at odds with a structural racism lens.

We, and organizations like ours, need to name and interrogate the mental models that may accidentally reinforce harmful norms of research. We need to ensure that we are aware of problematic norms and are making the strategic decision to work largely within them, rather than remaining unaware of them and allowing them to exert unnamed and unchecked influence. Naming the constraints and still pushing ourselves to do better can improve our ability to observe and describe our mental models and structures and their consequences. We are reflecting on where the project may have caused harm, and making plans to do better next time.

Urban's Racial Equity Framework provides some initial structure for this process of institutional self-reflection and interrogation. The fundamental orientation is that we will make Urban a more equitable organization by examining our institutional values, mental models, and culture and, from there, the systems and structures (e.g., policies, practices, and processes) that codify those. Namely, the Framework requires all staff to (1) continuously scrutinize institutional processes, norms, and behaviors; (2) grow the capacity of Urban teams and external partners to conduct equity-centered research; and (3) foster an environment of trust, learning, and accountability. The Racial Equity Framework is supported by detailed implementation and work plans as well as financial backing.

There are boundaries to what we can claim to know or see in this reflection process. Urban is a White-led, half-century old research organization. We are not experts on anti-racism. Even BIPOC researchers at Urban have benefited from the privileges of relatively elite education systems, living in relatively well-resourced neighborhoods and more. We have much to learn from the individuals who have lived within broken systems and who have spent lifetimes working to reform them through organizing, advocacy, research, practice, and policymaking. The boundaries established by our positionality also allow us to think deeply about what we know (and how), and offer insights to other organizations in comparable and adjacent places about ways we can reflect in order to change our practice. They also may limit our ability to see *all* the ways in which existing research structures could be changed to set up structural racism research for success.

Recommendations for Researchers and Funders

Below we include recommendations for how researchers can conceptualize their work and processes differently, and how funders can restructure calls for proposals and support research institutions to implement a shift toward more cross-cutting research on structural racism. This likely means dismantling hierarchies—between funders and researchers, between researchers at different stages of their career, between researchers and communities, and between methods (quantitative and qualitative). Such shifts require cross-project and cross-discipline infrastructure, training and professional development supports for experts of color from undergraduates to senior research (pipeline investments), and institutional and project-based community advisory boards.[16]

What Researchers Can Consider

Project Process and Structure

Our project cultivation and management experiment with these five projects suggested structures, supports, and requirements that research entities could offer to future projects in key stages.

---

[16] https://www.urban.org/research/publication/tools-and-resources-project-based-community-advisory-boards.

- **Target audience**: Each research team begins at a different starting point in terms of understanding structural racism and (in)equity, so every team cannot respond with the same depth or ease to a call for proposals on these interdisciplinary topics. This raises the question of who is the intended respondent to the call for proposals. One dimension relates to the applicant team's fluency with structural racism. By working with teams at different levels of fluency, cross-disciplinary entities like ORER, as well as the teams themselves, may see or understand the required growth areas to fluently analyze structural racism. An alternate option is to work with early adopters of structural racism frameworks and approaches, to generate proofs of concept that late adopters could follow in subsequent calls for proposals.

- **Solicitation**: Even before research teams apply for funding, they need working definitions of key concepts, exemplary papers from different disciplines, and models of mixed-methods research on structural racism. One way to deliver this support may involve a short workshop with assigned reading to prepare interested teams for the requirements of future projects like this. And while the offer of funding incentivizes research teams to pursue questions and learning they may not otherwise pursue, there needs to be ongoing structure and preparation so teams can successfully answer those questions and follow through on the structural racism analysis.

- **Conceptualization**: On the funder side, this involves considering what the process is as well as what the output or outcome is. For example, some calls for proposals may require engaging the community via a community advisory board to ensure that research is answering a necessary but missing question, rather than revisiting known disparities. An advisory board's presence might even encourage different kinds of teams to apply, knowing they would need to pursue this type of consultation and review in addition to technical review. Another aspect of process may relate to deepening team capacity to understand structural drivers at key milestones in the research process (e.g., background knowledge building, defining the problem/intended impact, question identification, determining methods and analysis plan, data collection, analysis, interpretation, dissemination).

- **Analysis plan**: In the proposal and then mid-project, more explanation of the selection of unit of analysis, modeling, and variable choices should be required to encourage more quantitative researchers to operationalize the ideas of structural racism more. Just as it is now common to have external technical review and pre-registration of analysis plans, reviewing for the analytic assumptions that may reinforce structural racism could become part of the study process. For example, if the unit of policy intervention or manipulation is at the system level, like the supply of services, then analysis may need to be at the system level and the individual decision-making level. Early level-setting showing that econometric or demographic methods can be applied in different ways can help researchers advance their methods expertise.

- **Draft**: At the drafting stage, research teams should be required to discuss in depth how their unit of analysis and analytic approach reflect the type of structural racism occurring in their specific policy system studied. Conceptual frameworks should also be thought through, to help teams understand that calling a policy race-neutral or saying there is no racially motivated intent behind the policy does not eliminate the need for a discussion of structural racism in adjacent policies and systems. Further, teams need support for a different kind of inference and discussion section on these interlocking systems, rather than overloading the limitations section of a paper in ways that undermine an argument about the presence of structural racism.

  This may involve requiring a race and equity expert as a coauthor and team member for each content team. This coauthor could be someone who has worked on creating new literature reviews, analytic frameworks, or measures of structural racism—all of which would deepen the integration of a structural lens. There is now a growing pool of researchers to draw from across education, public health, and other disciplines.

The project lifecycle model may be particularly well-suited to facilitating conversations about default values and norms of research and/or a specific discipline, how they can propagate inequity in the research process and outcomes, and how to intentionally reform them. For example, the milestone of defining the problem could be an opportunity to discuss whether research is what is actually needed to achieve the desired impact (for example, would more research revert to documenting disparities rather than generating solutions). Determining the research question and methods could be a prime moment for a conversation about normative methods, their shortcomings, and potential new approaches (community-engaged methods, participatory action research, systems science) that could be appropriate with the right capacity building, support, and partnership. Other norms that should be discussed in project teams include the role of the funder; research timeline; the definition of key concepts like quality, rigor, and success; and the set of incentives we use, at both the organization and field levels to encourage certain behaviors (e.g., equity vs. efficiency goals).

What Funders Can Consider

Resources and Supports

Provide pre-application trainings, workshops, and resource libraries to help researchers develop and implement proposals that effectively conceptualize structural racism and embrace antiracist practices. Recognizing that deepening one's understanding and capacity for framing structural solutions is a time-intensive and layered process, funders should consider multiphased approaches to support researchers. Even before the submissions of proposals, funders could provide trainings/workshops to help researchers frame their proposals through a structural racism lens. Though not all who participate will be selected, researchers could start conceptualizing their research questions and approach them in a manner that moves beyond disparities analysis.

For successful applicants, offer or require a period of reading and/or training for all members of the research team during an extended design and planning phase. Funders could provide an opportunity for selected researchers to learn during a pre-grant phase of reading and training, and then by starting a small pilot research project to learn through the process of doing. Not everyone will be fluent in structural racism by the time they start the project, but they can learn during the process. Given that familiarity with the available literature is so critical to understanding and contextualizing structural racism, funders should make available bibliographies and knowledge databases to researchers at the start of a project.

Enlist experts in race and equity research to offer coaching, support, and feedback at various points in the project life cycle. This could be a mandatory, or optional (but highly suggested), element of a call for proposals. The external reviewers and equity scholars were essential to keeping the papers focused on structural racism questions and analyses. The project teams appreciated the reviews they received and how they brought up issues that their internal team had not considered or framed in the same way.

Where feasible, develop communities of practice within and across grant programs. A community of practice may be necessary to help researchers navigate the inevitable and necessary discomfort. Pairing experienced equity researchers with applicants (starting at the application stage) can help them connect structural racism to their topical expertise (how does structural racism fit in/interact with how experts see and understand their area).

Funding and Time

Ensure that the size and duration of grants are sufficient for researchers to adopt new approaches, work across systems and disciplines, engage community actors, and iterate in response to feedback. Consider planning grants and/or funding for extensive learning and design phases.

Conducting research with a structural racism framing and approach is a departure for many researchers; thus, it's important to build in additional time to do the work. Researchers need time at the forefront of the project to better absorb and contextualize their research in the available literature. This is even more important because structural problems and structural solutions so often relate to multiple systems and policies, which could lie outside the researchers' domain. And these structural problems may have been identified in other literature and do not need to impose repeated burden on communities. Planning grants could give project teams time to map a broader, intersectional framework and incorporate structural racism considerations into the conceptualization and development of their ideas, research questions, and methods. They could also provide time to prepare teams with a baseline of literature, model papers, and analyses. A planning grant also could allow researchers to build relationships and conversations with community members who are participants or otherwise affected by a policy, to elicit potential drivers of structural inequities that researchers could then analyze.

The process of authentic reflection, examination, and community engagement also requires full (rather than expedited) institutional review board approval, which can take months. Abbreviated research timelines may hinder researchers' abilities to capture these necessary perspectives, thus replicating hierarchies that privilege researcher voices over those of participants.

For quantitative research, there needs to be more time to reconceptualize datasets, coding, and the use of variables, and to interrogate the methodological choices made. For qualitative research, time needs to be devoted to finding sites appropriate and ready to engage in structural-level conversations and to build trust within those communities. For example, in the substance use and child welfare projects, the teams needed time to iterate on interview protocols that may not immediately resonate with participants. Early engagement with participants may even lead to critical reshaping of operating definitions; such was the case for the transportation equity team, whose initial explanation for structural racism was, by their own reflection, too academic and did not resonate with the South Dallas community members.

How Researchers and Funders Can Work Together

Teams

Develop grant requirements, selection rubrics, and guidelines that foster collaboration, break down silos, and deemphasize seniority and credentials. Resources, trainings, and workshops should be aimed at more than the leader of a research project; they should include the broader team to shift the team culture and engage in more robust peer-to-peer dialogue. This also involves changes to develop career pathways, to bring in more scholars comfortable with doing this work. Cultivating a shift across fields to examine structural racism involves a different paradigm than other field-building and method-building efforts: it flips the hierarchy. This model requires shared leadership—senior scholars learning from their earlier career peers and providing opportunities, including dedicated funding, for early-career researchers to continue to build their skills and visibility in this work. It also involves disrupting the norm by which the most tenured individual leads, but instead gives this responsibility to the person with the most relevant frameworks. This new way of collaborating would be a natural outgrowth of recruitment and retention efforts for early-career researchers to bring new measures, frameworks, and research models. Researchers may need to see calls for proposals related to structural racism as opportunities to advance their own methodology, rather than as requirements to use someone else's.

In addition, funders should consider not just whether but also *how* teams include people who bring lived experience not only of interpersonal racism but also of the compounding challenges of barriers in housing, education, health and other systems. It is important that people with painful experiences of structural racism do not bear the burden of defining and redefining a field, and that they are part of a team where all members share some foundational knowledge and commitment to structural analysis.

Another consideration is whether to include members of the community as research team members, consultants, advisors or reviewers. Each presents a different opportunity for deepening understanding of how structural racism persists from policy to daily life. But each carries a different burden as well (discussed further below).

Concepts and Language

Provide guidance on definitions and conceptual frameworks in application materials. Calls could define structural racism and distinguish it from racial inequity (perhaps along the lines of what we did at the start of this chapter). Helping researchers and the community articulate structural racism as differences that arise or are maintained by historical or structural factors can help them add an explanatory layer (the why behind disparities) to their submission. When describing eligibility for funding, use language that indicates the grant is not merely a funding opportunity for analyzing racial variations.

Recommend and support the use of people-first, strength-oriented, and culturally competent language. Although there is not yet a universally held concept across the field for structural racism, there are some core principles related to people-first language, how variables are coded with certain labels, and how to frame or discuss histories and present situations informally and in research protocols. It is critical that researchers are mindful of their use of language around these ideas in every stage of their project, including their research questions, interview protocols, survey instruments, and so on. The definitions used need to connect with people's lived experiences in order to be useful in data collection. If survey instruments are still using deficit-oriented language and are misaligned with impacted community understanding, then response rates will be low, defeating the goal of using a validated instrument.

Methods

Support community engaged and participatory methods wherever possible. Involving community partners meaningfully is only possible when researchers have already developed trust with key actors. The two projects that were most successful at engaging community drew on relationships established from prior work and thoroughly integrated their perspectives into many aspects of the research design, data collection, and analysis, from definitions to interview questions to outcomes.

In particular, it may be worth exploring different forms of project-based Community Advisory Boards[17] as well as institutional or programmatic boards at major research institutions, as these standing boards can build the pipeline of community members who are fluent in research concepts and can advise on projects as needed. In addition, it may be worth setting criteria for what kinds of projects should have such a board, and how best to use them. True community engagement requires significant investments of time and money, and should not be used in reductive ways that merely check a box.

Use quantitative methods cautiously, not to expedite or narrow inquiry. If one treats structural racism as a cause with an effect on a key variable, that pattern may be easier to find in a single dataset. If one treats structural racism as a series of contextual factors, these may not be present in a single individual-level dataset but perhaps require merging multiple datasets and relying on multiple variables. Ask study teams to consider the datasets they are using, who is and is not represented, why that is, and what that means for inference.

Models generally focus on inputs rather than structures. Inputs can reflect disparities in terms of investments as well as outcomes; this is what typical multivariate regression analysis captures (and models race as a variable rather than racism as a system). In traditional (parametric) statistical modeling, one also needs to consider whether exploring structural racism requires conducting multiple hypothesis tests, rather than sticking to one or two pre-specified hypotheses. In addition, teams that aim to test whether differences between groups are statistically significant may want to consider whether the levels for significance need to be adjusted for different group sizes.

To go beyond a disparities analysis, one needs estimation models that reflect structures. Algorithms and simulations may be more able to account for existing and new patterns of policies by setting parameters and varying their values to reflect more or less intense prejudice or preference, and

---

[17] https://www.urban.org/research/publication/tools-and-resources-project-based-community-advisory-boards.

approximate some structural features of, say, a housing market. But they are still drawing on data that may have been collected to illuminate individual-level rather than structural features. These methodological approaches also bring other limitations and biases of past data collection and analyses. As Gee and Ford note, "Research on structural racism should not only focus on independent effects but also should address interactions among multiple forms of racism. Further, it is likely that forms of racism may reinforce one another, and efforts to dismantle one system may yield little effect without simultaneous efforts on another system...The study of single forms of racism would lead to an incomplete understanding and, potentially worse, biased estimates."[18] Teams should then specify how they are tackling this complexity, rather than disregarding it as beyond the scope of a paper.

Structural racism can be hard to capture in pure quantitative research, so mixed-methods research may be necessary rather than optional. Administrative or survey data tends to focus on individual or household attributes and outcomes. Qualitative data can better capture history, lived experience, and mechanisms—all of which are critical to understanding and applying a structural racism lens in research—but only if there is enough time and training.

Conclusion

The work discussed in this chapter affirmed that research organizations can help traditionally trained researchers adopt structural analysis on a project-by-project basis, while working toward a more substantive shift in how we conceptualize the purpose and products of research. Analyzing structural problems and making recommendations for structural solutions involves more than technical changes to research; it demands a major and comprehensive shift in the overall approach. In addition to incorporating more historical reflection and multi-system analysis, researchers need to design their work in ways that can inform and identify solutions, as opposed to merely naming problems.

Over time, research organizations and funders can catalyze change in the field both by investing intensively in early adopters and innovators and by helping larger numbers of established researchers deepen their

[18] Gilbert C. Gee and Chandra L. Ford. 2011. "Structural Racism and Health Inequities." *Du Bois Review: Social Science Research on Race* 8 (1): 115–132.

understanding of structural racism and bring more nuanced and informed structural perspectives to their work.

We encourage research institutions and funders to support action-oriented learning models like the project described in this chapter. With more time and resources, there may be greater potential to accelerate the learning and new ways of working necessary for lasting transformation.

6

Promoting Equity in the Justice System

Anthony Petrosino, Angelia Turner, Trevor Fronius, Trent Baskerville,
Pamela MacDougall, Ericka C. Muñoz, Danielle Munguia,
Leigha Puckett, and Cosette Lias

Introduction

The murder of George Floyd in May 2020 by members of the Minneapolis Police Department highlighted in a dramatic way the disparate experiences that Black, Indigenous, and People of Color (BIPOC) have when they encounter the justice system. The eight minutes and 46 seconds of video coverage of Floyd being murdered ignited protests and civil unrest across the United States. It also led to increased attention to addressing inequities and systemic racism across every aspect of society, most notably in the justice system.

For many decades, and long before the Floyd murder, the juvenile and adult justice systems in the United States have, however, grappled with racial (and ethnic) disparities in their outcomes. Findings from studies across policing (including police use of force), pretrial and bail decisions, sentencing, and corrections consistently indicate inequities in the experiences of BIPOC persons when compared to those of White people. In summary, BIPOC persons, on average, encounter the justice system more, receive harsher treatment when they encounter it, and experience worse outcomes when compared to their White counterparts.

When looking specifically at youth, US Department of Justice data on juvenile custodial institutions indicates that Native and Indigenous youth are twice as likely to be living in a secure facility as White youth, while Black youth are four times as likely. When viewed as an ethnicity, the rate of Latine youth residing in juvenile facilities is 42 percent higher than for White youth. Not surprisingly, these disparities exist across other systems that contribute to involvement in the juvenile justice system, particularly school discipline

Anthony Petrosino et al., *Promoting Equity in the Justice System*. In: *Research to Action*. Edited by: Claire Gibbons and Alonzo L. Plough, Oxford University Press. © Robert Wood Johnson Foundation (2026).
DOI: 10.1093/9780197819876.003.0007

and punishment. For example, Black and Native/Indigenous children are expelled at three times the rate of White students. Black girls are four times more likely than White girls to be suspended. Perhaps most alarmingly, these disparities begin in preschool with suspension and expulsion decisions.

If the involvement of the justice system had a benign effect on individuals, the impact of structural racism would be viewed as less alarming. But a long line of research studies documents the nefarious effects of system contact on individuals, particularly on their health. For example, at the most extreme, over 1,000 civilians were killed by police in 2022; data indicate that Black persons were three times more likely than Whites, during 2013–2022, to be killed in police encounters (Levin, 2023).

These are only some of the many data points that exist that underscore the racial and ethnic disparities evidenced in the justice system and their impact on BIPOC persons. Few would dispute these data. However, a critical question for policy and practice is not simply whether disparities exist but whether they can be mitigated. Are these the entrenched manifestations of a long history of systematic or institutional racism across many systems (health, education, justice, housing) that are impervious to intervention? Or can we reduce the impact of structural racism in the justice system and thereby improve the nation's health, particularly among BIPOC persons who are most in need of such mitigation?

This chapter, which describes the results of a comprehensive literature review and over 120 interviews with experts including those with lived justice system experience, provides a launching point. After underscoring the health importance of addressing structural racism in the justice system, we lay out our assumptions and methodology for the research described in herein. We then present results from the literature and interviews to define structural racism, what racial groups are most impacted, where it is most manifested in the system, data evidencing structural racism and what information and research gaps exist, and how we can best mitigate its negative health effects.

The Health Importance of Addressing Structural Racism in the Justice System

There are many reasons to implement strategies to mitigate the impact of structural racism in the justice system. Investments that promote such strategies could lead to improvements in the public's health, particularly within

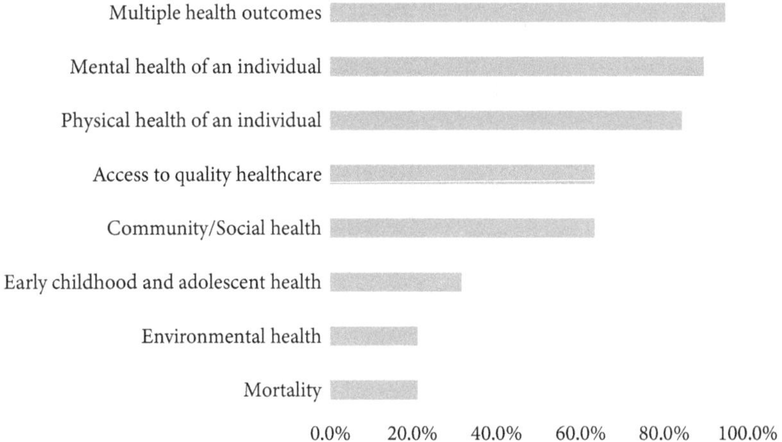

Figure 6.1 Percentage of reports mentioning specific health outcomes, by type

populations most impacted by the justice system. Numerous studies have documented the negative impacts that encounters with the justice system have on physical, mental, and behavioral health (e.g., Esposito et al. 2017). During our literature review task, we identified studies that examined a wide range of health outcomes from interaction with the justice system (Figure 6.1).

Some of these outcomes are immediate, such as the consequences of police violence against BIPOC citizens that results in injury or death (e.g., mortality or physical health). Some may be longer-term, such as the mental and physical health impacts of incarceration policies. To the extent that these policies are distributed disparately, the health outcomes will also be disparate.

For example, Bovell-Ammon and colleagues (2021) discuss a cohort study that followed participants for over 40 years and reported that incarceration was disproportionately experienced by non-Hispanic Black persons; they also experienced a 65 percent higher mortality rate, indicating a potential relationship between incarceration, racial disparities, and lower life expectancy. Mortality was not associated with incarceration in non-Black individuals. The impacts of incarceration extend beyond the person incarcerated as well. Morsy and Rothstein (2016) highlight that children of incarcerated fathers are 51 percent more likely to suffer from anxiety, 43 percent more likely to suffer from depression, and 72 percent more likely to suffer from post-traumatic stress disorder.

Assumptions

The research discussed in this chapter was guided by several assumptions. First, we did not undertake an exercise to "prove" the existence of structural racism in the justice system. We assumed that structural racism exists. Scholarly treatises, journalistic inquiries, and personal accounts have documented the long history of racism and its influence on the justice system, including, the creation of laws (Banaji et al. 2021), the disparate actions of police and other justice system actors (Gilbert & Ray, 2016), and the deep disparities in the justice system, particularly when comparing outcomes for BIPOC persons to White persons (Braveman et al. 2022).

Second, we did not attempt to parse out the contribution of structural racism in systems outside of the justice system. Many systems are intertwined, and BIPOC persons may pay an enormous price in the justice system because of structural racism in economics and labor, poor education, housing, and health care. Although structural racism in education, housing, labor, wealth accumulation, economic mobility, health care, and every other facet of American life is also well discussed, our focus here is on what we can do to specifically mitigate the deleterious impact of structural racism in the justice system.

Finally, we use White persons as the reference group, as do the bulk of research studies, for which to compare the greater involvement in the system of BIPOC persons. We do not try to explain why Asians, if presented as a monolithic racial group, have *lower* justice system involvement rates than Whites, if also presented as a monolithic racial group.

Methods

Literature Review

Our literature search focused exclusively on documents that discussed structural racism in the justice system. To be eligible for review, the document had to focus on the United States and, to be most relevant to the current policy context, published or available since 2010.

Our searches utilized *Criminal Justice Abstracts*, *Google*, and *Google Scholar* and relied upon different iterations of broad search terms related to structural racism in the justice system (e.g., combined searches of "structural racism" or "systemic racism" with "justice system" or "criminal justice"). We examined over 4,000 potential resources and determined that 83 were relevant to this project and are summarized here. Information from the documents was then coded and captured into an Excel spreadsheet that paralleled the categories in the interview protocol highlighted in the next section.

Key Stakeholder Interviews

As of January 2023, we have completed interviews with 123 key stakeholders. These interview participants were intentionally selected to represent diverse roles (e.g., policymaker, researcher, etc.), demographic backgrounds (gender identity and race), and geographic locations (located in several different states). Our sample includes justice system personnel including judges and lawyers, federal and state policy makers, reentry advocates, mental health professionals, academic and research experts, and current and former justice-impacted individuals. Overall, approximately 20 percent of our interviewees were justice-impacted individuals; just over two-thirds of the interview sample were persons of color, with the majority of those being African American/Black; the sample spanned across 21 different states and the District of Columbia; and the majority identified as female (approximately 60 percent).

Our interview protocol takes approximately 1 hour and was designed to be broad to elicit participants' views but structured to permit classification of participant responses into major themes. Each interview was conducted virtually by Zoom, included a notetaker when possible, and was recorded with permission. Like the documents retrieved for the literature review, our team coded the information from the interviews into thematic categories, as organized below.

Findings

Defining Structural Racism

Finding a single agreed upon definition of structural racism as it relates to the justice system is an elusive task. Structural racism is a term that is often used interchangeably with systemic racism, historical racism, and institutional racism. But across documents and interviews, there was a clear understanding that structural racism represents something more powerful and built in than any individual actor's racism. As one interviewee stated, "it is the racism in the system that persists even if everyone in the system is neutral" and leads to disparate outcomes because of what has been built into the system through law, history, policies, and practices.

Structural racism has been broadly defined in the literature as historical racial discrimination that has been intertwined into societal institutions and structures, resulting in cyclical, inequitable systems such as the criminal justice system. As several interviewees discussed, the United States has a history of violence and racial inequity that was built into the criminal justice system at the very beginning. Laws were often created and enforced, for example, to protect the subjugation of Native/Indigenous and African American populations (e.g., "Jim Crow" laws). As one interviewee pointed out, it has morphed into today's practices which conflate "race with criminality and dangerousness." As another stakeholder noted, "this kind of [racist] ideology informs a lot of the ways in which laws, policies, and practices are written, implemented, and carried out to perpetuate a type of racial inequality."

These inequities mostly manifest themselves as disparities in treatment at each stage of the system, from policing to reentry into the community. For example, multiple stakeholders noted the disproportionate rates in people of color in juvenile halls and prisons relative to their White counterparts who committed similar crimes. It appears, as one interviewee stated, that "Black and Brown males that are currently incarcerated for very similar charges as their [White] counterparts get the majority of the time inside of these systems. When we look at just the whole political structure, on the outside of the prison you find that majority of resources go to communities of other races other than the Black and Brown communities." Another example in which this bias is portrayed is in the inequity within police surveillance and presence in communities. For instance, one stakeholder concluded that "Black folks are not possessing weapons at a higher rate or possessing other types of controlled substances at a higher rate. It means that there's a greater access; there's greater access to the Black community, which results in more arrests within the community."

Because structural racism exists within every facet of the justice system, the deleterious effects are compounded the further entrenched individuals and populations become within it.

Racial Groups Referenced

The data from both the literature and the interviews converged in identifying Black/African Americans as the group most impacted by structural racism. A few interviewees also expanded beyond Black Americans to discuss Native/Indigenous Americans and Asian Americans, including Vietnamese and Cambodians. The complexity of defining what is a racial group was underscored by both the literature and some interviewees identifying Latine persons (often identified as an ethnic and not racial category) as a people that have been impacted by structural racism. Literature also referenced other non-racial groups of people, including persons with low income, LGBTQ+ persons, and individuals with disabilities.

Part of the Justice System Manifested

Many interviewees identified policing/law enforcement as the part of the system in which structural racism is most evidenced. Some interviewees discussed this in the context of "initial system contact," with structural racism compounded for the individual as they progressed through each phase of the system. Most of the literature we retrieved highlighted that structural racism manifests across the justice system, with law enforcement and the courts being the most cited components (Figure 6.2). Although "victims" is not a specific component of the system, how crime victims are treated and what services they receive are intertwined with the traditional justice system components of policing, courts, and corrections.

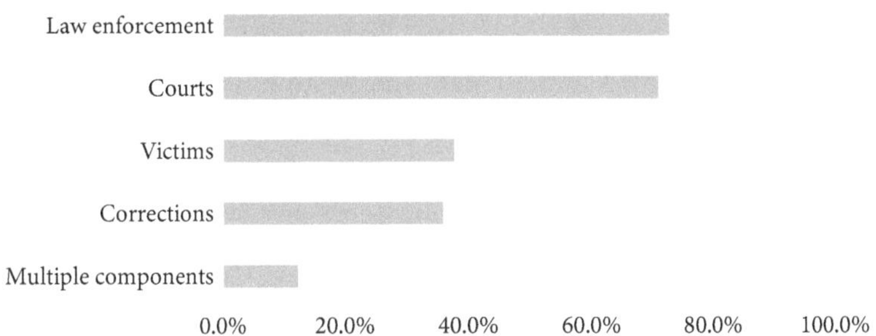

Figure 6.2 Prevalence of structural racism across justice system components

The literature identified major themes as it related to structural racism and observed disparities and unfairness in the justice system. For example:

Harsh policing tactics (e.g., use of force, stop and frisk) and over-surveillance in policing. For example, Duarte and colleagues (2020) explain that Black boys experience more frequent stops by the police on the street than do White boys (45 percent vs. 26 percent) with similar patterns observed among Black and White girls (18 percent vs 8 percent).

Disparities in arrests for low-level or less serious offenses. For example, Nellis (2021) describes arrests for low-level drug offenses that create disparate outcomes by race. Black and White individuals use and sell drugs at comparable levels, but Black people are nearly four times as likely as Whites to be arrested for drug offenses and two-and-a-half times as likely to be arrested for drug possession.

Wrongful convictions. Kovera (2019) explains that innocent Black people are three-and-a-half times more likely than innocent White people to be convicted of sexual assault, seven times more likely to be convicted of murder, and 12 times more likely to be convicted of drug crimes.

Mandatory sentencing and repeat offender laws. For example, Mauer and Ghandnoosh (2014) describe federal prosecutors as twice as likely to charge Black defendants relative to White defendants with offenses that carry mandatory minimum sentences. State prosecutors are also more likely to charge Black rather than similar White defendants under habitual offender laws.

Disproportionate access to health care while incarcerated. This was another place in which structural racism is manifested in the system, including differential diagnoses of mental health issues upon the start of a custodial sentence, and insufficient access for Black and Brown women to perinatal care. As an example, Nellis and colleagues (2016) indicate that African Americans tend to be diagnosed as schizophrenic disproportionately more often than Whites; the latter tend to be diagnosed as presenting depressive symptoms. The differences in diagnosis may reflect the cultural distance between African American persons who are incarcerated and the generally White personnel in psychological services positions and may result in a different assessment of the potential dangerousness of the incarcerated individual.

The interview data yielded similar feedback regarding examples of where in the justice system structural racism manifests itself. However, interviewees focused a lot of attention on law enforcement because encounters with police are usually the gateway for most people into the justice system. That initial arrest can lead to compounding impacts as the individual progresses through the formal system. In addition, encounters with the justice system can lead to the person being labeled a criminal, a danger, or a problem individual to be further monitored.

As highlighted in the literature, the over-policing and surveillance of Black and Brown communities can lead to more contact and arrests. A few interview participants highlighted the self-fulfilling prophecy of policing communities: law enforcement agencies find more crime in Black and Brown communities because of increased scrutiny and surveillance, and that "criminal danger" justifies even further resources being devoted to further police those communities, leading to the identification of "more crime" and more arrests. Interview participants also highlighted the increased risk for Black and Brown persons (particularly young men), as mentioned in the chapter's introduction, to be killed or injured by the police using deadly force.

Interview participants also highlighted the compounding impacts of structural racism through the formal justice system, after arrest. For example, Black and Brown defendants may be more likely to face harsher penalties, even if they accept plea bargains, than their White counterparts who committed the same offense and have a similar prior criminal history. Black and Brown defendants, particularly those from lower-income communities, are less likely to be able to afford a private attorney and therefore rely on the public criminal defender offices for representation. Public defenders are frequently understaffed and overworked, and they may push young Black and Brown persons to accept plea bargains that may not be much of a bargain and result in jail or prison time.

Interviewees also talked at great length about the heavy toll of incarceration on Black and Brown Americans. As mentioned above, the research on the deleterious impacts of incarceration on health is well established. Such incarceration often separates persons from their families and communities, sometimes to be housed in facilities located in rural and isolated areas and where corrections officers and administrators are from a different race and ethnic background. As discussed in the literature, interviewees also noted the disparate access to education and vocational training and to receiving adequate health care, particularly mental health services. These factors are compounded and result in a person who is more likely to return to the justice system upon release to the community.

Data Supporting the Role of Structural Racism

Our project identified that a wide range of data on disparities is used as evidence for structural racism. In the literature, studies often drew on official or administrative data to identify disparities across justice system events, including:

Health outcomes, including data on fatalities to examine racial disparities in being victimized by police violence. For example, Serchen and colleagues (2020) describe that Black men are two-and-a-half times more likely to be killed by law enforcement than White men, making law enforcement violence one of the leading causes of death for young men alongside accidents, suicide, homicide, heart disease, and cancer.

Data on justice involvement of Black youth. To illustrate, Mallett (2018) used arrest, referral to court, detainment, formal processing, and adjudication data to show disproportionate involvement at every stage of the juvenile justice process.

Population-level data on incarceration, parole violation, and revocation rates. Hetey and Eberhardt (2018) emphasize that only 13 percent of the US population at the time of their study was African American, yet they comprised nearly 40 percent of the nation's inmates. Black men are incarcerated in state or federal prison at a rate six times that of White men. During their lifetime, one in three African American males can expect to be imprisoned compared with one in 17 White males.

Court data on prosecutorial discretion and plea bargaining. As an example, Kovera (2019) describes in the case of charging that racial differences begin when individuals are young, with prosecutors more likely to charge Black than White youth as adults under some circumstances, depriving them of the more lenient and rehabilitation-based treatment they would receive in the juvenile justice system.

For interviewees, findings from studies of disparity in the system were also cited as evidence of structural racism. Some of the data used as evidence of structural racism across literature and interviews included: data on injuries and death due to police violence; administrative statistics indicating the overexposure to the justice system at various points from arrest through incarceration; and longitudinal data on imprisonment and physical and mental health. A few interviewees pointed out that these data are often used by White supremacists and others with racist attitudes to depict Black and Brown persons as having character flaws and being prone to criminality.

Most striking was how such a wide range of data almost universally pointed to deep disparities between Black persons and their White counterparts on every dimension, including:

- the percentage of each racial group in decision-making positions;
- officer assignments to neighborhoods (for example, Black and Brown officers receiving the most "dangerous" crime area to patrol);
- a wide range of sentencing data (including length of time sentenced, percentage of defendants that had adequate legal defense, bond amounts, plea and diversion offers, parole grant rates, percentage of children being tried as adults);
- data on incarceration (including prison and jail populations compared to general populations, healthcare and medications being provided (whether they are sedatives), number of assaults in prison, rates of restraints, rates of seclusion); and
- data from other social institutions (e.g., discipline records in schools).

Data and Research Gaps

Lack of data and data collection that limit the ability to adequately measure the extent of structural racism in the justice system were at the forefront of the literature review findings. This was elaborated on by several interviewees, who stated that there is a "wealth of data" but turning information into "knowledge" that is actionable is a challenge because the organization and accessibility of that data vary widely. As interviewees noted, not all desired data that could shed light on structural racism and disparities are collected, reported, or analyzed. For example, as the literature points out, despite the disproportionate and often devastating impact of police use of deadly force in Black/Brown and marginalized communities, there is insufficient information on this, including physical and mental health harm outcomes, and the racial and other demographic characteristics of the law enforcement officer and persons involved.

Even available data are not easily found and are fragmented across different agencies, websites, and systems. Different agencies may capture race differently (e.g., police and court data may differ), making it difficult to compare data across systems. For some systems, they may provide options when collecting data that lists "Hispanic" as a race versus an ethnicity, adding to the confusion. A common issue across systems is that data are often not connected, and without a common identifier, it is impossible to link data for specific individuals. Some of the literature highlighted that correctional populations are often not included in large, national health surveys; this skews the "national sample" results, given the generally poorer health of incarcerated persons. It also misses an opportunity to learn more about the health of individuals in custody.

Several interview participants highlighted our need for qualitative research to explain the quantitative research into disparities. Incorporating people with lived experience into the research is also important; when people with lived experience are connected to the research on incarceration, it leads to a more accurate and deeper analysis than what researchers analyzing data will be able to do. One interviewee stated, "I think you guys are doing it now [filling a research gap] by talking to folks that are directly impacted from the community." Several interviewees mentioned a need for more narratives and participatory data in research to understand and mitigate structural racism in the justice system. This would involve asking how people are feeling and how they are being impacted, and data beyond the numbers reported by government agencies.

There is also a need for more research on what works. Getting quality data to assess which programs are best serving people impacted by the justice system could help mitigate some of the effects of structural racism, particularly if effective programs could be scaled up across communities and jurisdictions. The literature highlighted the lack of rigorous studies, such as randomized controlled trials, to better ascertain the impact of custody/incarceration. Other research gaps that interviewees mentioned were studies on the social, emotional, or academic effects on children of incarcerated parents; studies on incarcerated women; and studies on intergenerational trauma and neighborhood impacts. Moreover, few studies examine how the life-course timing, or duration/dosage of criminal justice encounters, affects physical and mental health.

Addressing Structural Racism and Improving Health

In this section, we summarize the literature review and interview data on what authors and interviewees recommended as strategies for mitigating the impact of structural racism and improving health. Their recommendations were focused more generally on what improvements can be made to society or the system, or what broader US policies were needed. Given the complexity and breadth and depth of structural racism in the United States, including the justice system, it was predictable that most suggested strategies would also be far-reaching and broad.

One clear path from the literature review is that efforts need to be undertaken to improve the evidence base through advocacy for and use of mandated measures of racism that include openly available disaggregated data in policing practices, courts, and corrections (including jail systems). Efforts to improve data, as some literature advocated, also need to focus on the availability, quality, and accessibility of data on correctional health care quality. Such data would help us better understand what services persons in custody are receiving, the quality of those services, the outcomes from those services, and how they may differ by the race of the treated person.

As highlighted in the section on data and research gaps, there is a need for careful studies to better understand the use and impact of strategies designed to mitigate disparities in the justice system. For example, what is the value of having "racial impact statements" in justice reform efforts in a jurisdiction? What are the impacts when a city declares racism a public health emergency? Several interview participants also advocated for closer collaboration between communities and research entities on studies.

Not surprisingly, given the negative impacts of contact for Black and Brown persons with the justice system, the literature and interview data converge on advocating for strategies that reduce the opportunity for such contact and further progression into the formal justice system. This includes diversionary alternatives at each stage of the juvenile and adult justice process to provide culturally informed and equitable mental health treatment and other supports outside of the formal system. Interviewees also recommended providing greater access to culturally competent mental health treatment, whether as a diversionary alternative or outside of the justice system altogether. At least one interviewee discussed the attention needed to address the "school to prison pipeline" or the flow of students, by referral, who commit disciplinary offenses into the formal juvenile justice system.

Because law enforcement is for most persons their most common point of contact with the justice system, it is not surprising that several recommendations from the literature and interviewees were specific to addressing police behavior and organizations. A few interview participants advocated for a "public safety" emphasis that does not rely solely on police to be the first responders to every situation in a community. Other interviewees talked about the need for law enforcement organizations to change from paramilitary structures and embrace reforms that include fairness and transparency at all stages of their work.

Another bracket of strategies from the literature and interview data centers on community support and resources. A few interviewees, for example, strongly advocated for an infusion of funds into certain communities, including job-training programs to "level the playing field in employment." As indicated by our literature review, community-based organizations are needed that are close to the ground and can support children and families of color experiencing the negative health outcomes that result from the incarceration of parents or over-policing in their communities. Interview participants also stressed the need for community programs that would increase the engagement and voice of citizens in those communities. The infusion of resources into disadvantaged communities, including expanded mentorship opportunities, financial literacy training, youth apprenticeship programs, access to safe recreation and proper nutrition were also recommended by interview participants.

Data from the interviews also lent support to strategies that could limit the impact of structural racism in existing laws and policies. For example, interviewees recommended that certain low-level and non-violent offenses be decriminalized to limit the formal justice system's involvement in responding to the behavior. Another set of recommendations has to do with limiting the disparity at the sentencing stage to ensure that race plays no role in influencing the type of punishment a person receives for a given offense. The stigma of a felony record, particularly when it comes to reentry and employment, also must be dealt with to expand work opportunities for persons leaving custodial facilities and reentering communities to live. At least one interviewee advocated for the closing of "private prisons" as they lead to more abuses of Black and Brown persons in custody.

Some of the literature also advocated for improvements to systems that would advance the health of those caught up in it, which would greatly impact Black and Brown persons, given their disproportionate involvement in the justice system. For example, the literature discussed the challenges of obtaining transportation or having finances to obtain good-quality health care for those reentering communities after incarceration. Community health centers were advocated in some reports as a way of providing a local, one-stop place during reentry to meet those needs. Several interview participants also advocated for more post-incarceration support during reentry. Another area for improvement that some literature stressed is the health care conditions within custodial facilities, with a special focus on providing prenatal healthcare for women who are incarcerated and access to evidence-based addiction treatment. Several interview participants strongly recommended greater access to effective substance abuse and trauma-informed treatment programs while under correctional or community supervision as a strategy to reduce the impact of structural racism.

Another set of recommendations, generally stemming from the interview data, focused on addressing the implicit and explicit racial biases of persons in justice policy and practice decision-making positions. This would include hiring and promoting a more diverse workforce, expanding diversity, equity, and inclusion (DEI) programs within jurisdictions, developing training modules for staff specific to understanding and addressing structural racism, and, to impact potential staff at the earliest inception, teaching critical race theory and the justice system to students in K-12 educational settings.

Recommendations to Philanthropy

The data from our literature review and interviews certainly help shape our recommendations to philanthropy. This is coupled, however, with our understanding that foundations are not governmental entities and have no authority over the justice system. With that in mind, we offer the following recommendations on how foundations can leverage their own resources to potentially mitigate the impact of structural racism in the justice system on health.

Before Law or Policy Is Enacted

Policies and laws are often enacted in jurisdictions without consideration as to how they may lead to disparate outcomes. Once laws or policies are enacted, they can cause great harm and often take considerable effort and time to roll back or repeal. Philanthropy could fund a pilot with an interested state jurisdiction that would put in place an equity review mechanism. The purpose of this racial equity review mechanism is to ensure that there is adequate input on potential racial impact and other disparities that may result from the considered legislation or policy. The structure of this racial equity review could be modeled after medical organizations that get the input of multiple medical ethicists on the ethics of health care practices. The mechanism could involve a Task Force of experts and community members, or a specific Chief Equity Officer in Justice position that requires "sign off" (or is provided an opportunity to weigh in) on proposed legislation. Such a review mechanism can also be used to examine existing laws to determine if revisions are needed to limit disparities. To the extent that such disparities can be reduced by changing or halting justice legislation or policy that sets in stone or exacerbates the impact of structural racism, public health potentially can be improved.

At the Police Contact Stage

The initial police contact is often the starting point for engagement with the system and leads to a compounding impact of structural racism at every subsequent stage (courts, corrections, etc.). Given the research that demonstrates harmful physical and mental health effects of system contact, philanthropy could support, perhaps as a coalition along with the US Department of Justice, a call for proposals for implementing and studying diversionary alternatives. This could be diversion of initial calls to other non-police agencies (e.g., social workers or mental health professionals), or diversion programs that can move individuals from the formal system to non-punitive treatment or other alternatives. Such diversionary programs, if effective, can mitigate the impact of structural racism in the justice system by preventing it from being introduced, reducing opportunities for negative police-civilian interactions (including death and injury from use of force), and from compounding with interest at later system stages, thereby improving the health of individuals and communities.

Another option for philanthropy is to fund a project to conduct a policy scan and identify innovative practices in diversionary alternatives or different approaches by jurisdictions to handling public safety calls. Many such innovations are being undertaken in the community, and many of these have not been evaluated. Innovative approaches that were identified in the policy scan could then become the prime candidates for evaluations funded as advocated above.

After Experiencing a Violent Crime

Crimes, especially violent crimes, result in significant losses for victims and their families, including health care costs, loss of employment and wages, and the need to obtain mental health counseling and treatment. At the federal level, via the US Department of Justice's Office of Victim Assistance, the Crime Victim Fund has been established to provide support for victims as they try to recover physically, mentally, and financially from the impact of an offense. However, research shows racial and other disparities in who accesses and receives these funds; persons most disproportionately impacted by crime are not taking up this support.

Philanthropy can investigate whether it can leverage its resources and influence to encourage uptake of these funds, particularly by minority and lower-income persons, who are also at greatest risk of violent crime victimization. One mechanism that could be used is to support community-based intermediaries who can work in marginalized neighborhoods to increase awareness of these funds and encourage their uptake by the very folks who could benefit the most from them.

During the Custodial Sentence

The lack of equity in health care conditions within jails and prisons was supported by both the interviews and the literature review. This was particularly true for women who are incarcerated, especially women who are pregnant, and for those suffering from drug addictions. Access to adequate treatment is inequitable, and there is a lack of data and knowledge about the effectiveness of such treatment. Philanthropy can support and convene an expert task force to better understand health care in custodial facilities. This task force would be comprised of policy, research, and practice experts, including those with lived experience in the system. Such a task force would solicit research presentations, expert testimony, and public comment so that it can form recommendations in this space.

One possible avenue is to fund the National Academies of Science, Engineering and Medicine,[1] by its Committee on Law and Justice, to bear the responsibility of convening and implementing such a task force. This is something the National Institute of Justice and the US Department of Education have both done several times in the past to get a representative group of experts to look at a specific topic, conduct a comprehensive review of it, and issue a non-partisan, consensus report. These National Academies panel reports are often the most trusted documents in Congress and among other policymakers because they have been through a rigorous sensing process. There is precedent for philanthropic support for National Academies panels; several foundations helped sponsor the panel on *Reducing Racial Inequalities in the Justice System.*

At the Reentry Stage after Incarceration

Most persons sentenced to a custodial term are going to leave a prison or jail facility to return to their communities. The health outcomes of persons who leave prisons and other facilities to reenter society are often substandard, often due to lack of access to quality health care, both while in custody and in reentry. Upon reentry to the community, the formerly incarcerated person faces significant challenges to obtaining employment, getting reliable transportation, and having income to support their health care needs. Philanthropy can support a special initiative to fund and pilot a transitional health center in a community to determine if this is a program model that can reduce poor health outcomes among reentry clients, many of whom are from racial and ethnic minority groups.

Recommendations Relevant to Data, Research, and Evaluation

Philanthropy can make investments, as we just recommended in the preceding section, to promote more effective policies, identify innovative strategies, and investigate current practice to mitigate the impact of structural racism in the justice system, thereby improving public health. Another type of investment that it can make, and which some foundations have a history of

---

[1] WestEd and its JPRC do not have any existing relationship with the National Academies, although several WestEd employees, including lead author Anthony Petrosino, have served on Committees and panels.

making, is to promote better quality data and more research and evaluation to increase our knowledge about the impact of structural racism and how we might counter it.

Evaluating Initiatives to Reduce Disparities in the Justice System

Although there is substantial research on racial disparities in justice, there is comparatively little research on "what works" to reduce such disparities. Although the National Institute of Justice has recommitted to funding studies in this area, its annual budget usually means that only a handful of studies can be funded each year. Philanthropic organizations can promote a funding solicitation for more studies to fill this gap. This can be a more targeted Request for Proposals (RFP) for such studies as they relate to the justice system. One intervention that could be studied, for example, is the impact of racial impact statements on criminal justice reform initiatives. A requirement from studies funded under this initiative is that it must involve community partners and persons with lived experience, include a plan for active involvement of those partners and persons with lived experience, and be staffed by a diverse evaluation team.

Addressing Data Issues Relevant to Structural Racism in the Justice System

The problem of structural racism cannot be addressed unless those instances in which clear disparities exist are identified. Philanthropy can improve data by advocating for the use of indicators that include openly available and disaggregated data by race on justice practices in policing, prosecution, courts, and corrections (including local jails). As previously highlighted, a particular need is to create data to allow for analyses of correctional health care quality, who is getting access to high-quality services, and whether these services are being delivered equitably.

Foundations may consider funding a justice data-focused organization, such as *Equal Measures for Justice* (https://www.measuresforjustice.org/),[2] to specifically advocate for improved data in this area. This is a model used by

---

[2] WestEd and the JPRC have no relationship or connection to Measures for Justice and are using that organization as an example of an intensive data-focused team with expertise in justice that could serve in this role.

the Gates Foundation in its funding of the *Data Quality Campaign* (https://dataqualitycampaign.org/); its efforts led to considerable advancement in longitudinal databases in education and an increase in their reliability and use in decision-making. In short, the organization's work could consist of publications to highlight challenges and strategies to overcome them, and advocacy in government circles to promote funding to improve data systems (such as what happened in education with the federal State Longitudinal Database funding from the Institute of Education Sciences) and highlight how improved data systems benefit decision making and the public's health.

There are also no regularly collected data on police-citizen encounters. Given the role of police violence in citizen health, and that these encounters are the entry point into the system for some citizens, it is important to capture these data. One possible solution is to expand the current US Department of Justice's Police-Public Contact Survey (PPCS) to examine citizens' perceptions of police behavior and responses during police encounters. This is the responsibility of the Bureau of Justice Statistics (BJS); advocacy by philanthropy could influence BJS to adopt that as part of its agenda.

Limitations

Our research relied upon a comprehensive literature review and interviews, conducted up to this point, with over 120 stakeholders. Although care was taken to be as representative as possible in our sample, it is possible that our literature and participant sample were biased. For example, our discussion here was very dominated by disparities between African American persons versus White persons in the justice system. Although disparities for Native/Indigenous persons were mentioned, they received comparatively scant attention. This may be a function of the focus of the articles we retrieved as well as the people we interviewed. Very few of our interview participants or the writers of documents we retrieved, for example, were Native/Indigenous or familiar with the data on this population, and that likely influenced how they viewed structural racism in the US justice system. Consequently, it is possible that we missed gathering information that could have informed specific recommendations that could mitigate the harmful effects of structural racism experienced by Native/Indigenous populations. However, the recommendations we offer were not specific to African Americans, and if implemented with good fidelity, could mitigate the impact of structural racism as experienced by African Americans, Native/Indigenous, and other racial groups.

References

Banaji, M.R., Fiske, S.T., & Massey, D.S. (2021). Systemic racism: Individuals and interactions, institutions and society. *Cognitive Research* 6: 82.

Bovell-Ammon, B. J., Xuan, Z., Paasche-Orlow, M. K., & LaRochelle, M. R. (2021). Association of incarceration with mortality by race from a national longitudinal cohort study. *JAMA Network Open* 4(12). https://jamanetwork.com/journals/jamanetworkopen/fullarticle/2787436

Braveman, P.A., Arkin, E., Proctor, D., Kauh, T., & Holm, N. (2022). Systemic and structural racism: Definitions, examples, health damages, and approaches to dismantling. *Health Affairs* 41(2): 171–178.

Duarte, C.D.P., Salas-Hernandez, L., & Griffin, J.S. (2020). Policy determinants of inequitable exposure to the criminal legal system and their health consequences among young people. *American Journal of Public Health* 110: S43–S49.

Esposito, M.H., Lee, H., Hicken, M.T., Porter, L.C., & Herting, J.R. (2017). The consequences of contact with the criminal justice system for health in the transition to adulthood. *Longitudinal Life Course Studies* 8(1): 57–74.

Gilbert, K.L. & Ray, R. (2016). Why police kill black males with impunity: Applying public health critical race praxis (PHCRP) to address the determinants of policing behaviors and "justifiable" homicides in the USA. *Journal of Urban Health* 93(Suppl 1): 122–140.

Hetey, R.C. & Eberhardt, J.L. (2018). The numbers don't speak for themselves: Racial disparities and the persistence of inequality in the criminal justice system. *Current Directions in Psychological Science* 27(3): 183–187.

Kovera, M. B. (2019). Racial disparities in the criminal justice system: Prevalence, causes, and search for solutions. *Journal of Social Issues* 75(4): 1139–1164.

Levin, S. (2023). "It never stops": Killings by US police reach record high in 2022. *The Guardian.* January 6. https://www.theguardian.com/us news/2023/jan/06/us police killings-record-number-2022.

Mallett, C.A. (2018). Disproportionate minority contact in juvenile justice: Today's, and yesterday's, problems. *Criminal Justice Studies* 31(3): 230–248.

Mauer, M. & Ghandnoosh, N. (2014). *Incorporating racial equity into criminal justice reform.* Washington, DC: The Sentencing Project. https://www.safetyandjusticechallenge.org/wp-content/uploads/2015/05/incorporating-racial-equity-into-criminal-justice-reform.pdf.

Morsy, L. & Rothstein, R. (2016). *Mass incarceration and children's outcomes: Criminal justice policy is education policy.* Washington, DC: Economic Policy Institute. https://www.epi.org/publication/mass-incarceration-and-childrens-outcomes/.

Nellis, A. (2021). *The color of justice: Racial and ethnic disparity in state prisons.* Washington, DC: The Sentencing Project. https://www.sentencingproject.org/publications/color-of-justice-racial-and-ethnic-disparity-in-state-prisons/.

Nellis, A., Greene, J., & Mauer, M. (2016). *Reducing racial disparity in the criminal justice system.* Washington, DC: The Sentencing Project. https://www.sentencingproject.org/wp-content/uploads/2016/01/Reducing-Racial-Disparity-in-the-Criminal-Justice-System-A-Manual-for-Practitioners-and-Policymakers.pdf.

Serchen, J., Doherty, R., Atiq, O., & Hilden, D. (2020). Racism and health in the United States: A policy statement from the American College of Physicians. *Annals of Internal Medicine* 173: 556–557.

RESEARCH MEETS COMMUNITY REALITIES: ACTION AND ENGAGEMENT TO CONFRONT STRUCTURAL RACISM

Section III, taking action: Empowered communities, responsive research recognizes the need to translate scholarship, broadly defined, into inclusive strategies with transformative potential. A full-throated commitment to community-informed research designed to eliminate racial inequities is long overdue. Approaches that cross disciplines and sectors, pay special attention to implicit bias, and translate knowledge into practice are among the essential tools for disrupting structural racism. The three chapters in this part offer strategies for overhauling the criminal justice system, cultivating the healing power of Indigenous traditions, combatting the dehumanization of Black bodies, and addressing climate change at the community level.

Chapter 7: Overcoming Colonial Subjugation, Privileging Indigenous Health tracks the historical trauma of American Indians and Alaskan Natives following European contact. By exploring the harms of reservation structures, forced relocation, dispossession, assimilation, and boarding school abuses, this chapter exposes the devastation caused by colonial policies. But resilience, resistance, and well-being also emerge, shifting the narrative from pathology to promise. Honoring the culture, knowledge, worldview, and wellness practices embedded in Indigenous cultures, and empowering these original inhabitants with financial and political support, fosters revitalized communities. Their physical, mental, and emotional health depend on self-governance, a spiritual connection to the land, and thriving intergenerational relationships.

Chapter 8: Black Bodies, Black Health: Disrupting Structural Racism Through Humanistic and Social Science Research confronts the assumption that White bodies are the norm, with Black bodies represented only in the context of disorder and disease. The resulting dehumanization helps to perpetrate the myth that biological differences can be explained by race, undermines women's reproductive well-being, and enables unethical medical experimentation. The humanities and social sciences provide the intellectual framework for understanding the structures and systems that promote a distorted cultural imagination of disease. Recognizing their historical origins, and how they have been carried through to modern discourse creates an opportunity to disrupt the pathways that have undermined wellness.

Chapter 9: Centering Health Equity and Community Voice in Climate Change acknowledges the disproportionate health impact of a warming planet on communities of color while emphasizing that genuine progress is not possible without addressing structural racism more broadly. The existential threats of climate change are compounded by biased environmental policy and the inequities that reflect racial segregation, generational poverty, economic disinvestment, and violence. Four primary power-influencing structures were identified through a community-informed process of inquiry: electoral justice, economic justice, power and decisionmaking authority, and narrative. To make their most effective contributions, enlightened funders must consider their own internal systems and culture, reimagine their conception of evidence, build trust, and share power.

7

Overcoming Colonial Subjugation, Privileging Indigenous Health

Rachel E. Wilbur, (Tolowa Nation/Chetco descent), Miigis B. Gonzalez, (Lac Courte Oreilles Ojibwe), Stephanie Russo Carroll, (Ahtna/Dene-Native Village of Kluti Kaah), Jill M. Doerfler, (White Earth Anishinaabe), Jillian Fish, (Tuscarora Nation of the Haudenosaunee Confederacy), Michelle Kahn-John, (Diné), Victoria M. O'Keefe, (Cherokee Nation/Seminole Nation), Myra Parker, (Mandan/Hidatsa/Cree), Thomas D. Sequist, (Taos Pueblo), Carly Chiwiwi, (Pueblo of Laguna), Tonya M. Connor, (Arapaho descent), Liz Contreras, Tara L. Maudrie, (Sault Ste Marie Tribe of Chippewa Indians), Melissa L. Walls, (Couchiching First Nation/Bois Forte Anishinaabe descent), and Joseph P. Gone, (Aaniiih-Gros Ventre, Fort Belknap Indian Community)

Introduction

American Indian and Alaska Native (AIAN) citizens of the United States, as demonstrated by their very existence today, are resilient peoples. AIAN reservation, rural, and urban communities are heirs to rich cultural assets that have survived and thrived against all odds; to relational worldviews that promote belonging, connectedness, and well-being; and to resourceful innovations that have ensured persistence, survival, and success in the wake of colonial subjugation. Nevertheless, AIANs also experience documented health inequities that have taken a profound toll. Whether expressed as disproportionately high rates of physical (e.g., cancer, diabetes, heart disease, hepatitis, obesity) or mental and behavioral health (e.g., substance abuse, posttraumatic stress, suicide) disorders, these conditions reappear over time and across generations in our communities. They lead AIANs to experience the highest rates of premature mortality in the nation. It is commonplace to attribute these inequities to social and structural determinants of health

Rachel E. Wilbur et al., *Overcoming Colonial Subjugation, Privileging Indigenous Health.* In: *Research to Action.* Edited by: Claire Gibbons and Alonzo L. Plough, Oxford University Press. © Robert Wood Johnson Foundation (2026). DOI: 10.1093/9780197819876.003.0008

such as poverty, segregation, discrimination, and restricted access to educational and employment opportunities. *Yet this legacy of disadvantage—long described as oppression and discrimination, and more recently characterized as historical trauma and structural racism—was no accident of history, but rather was orchestrated by Euro-American settlers through centuries of savage dispossession and subjugation of Indigenous Peoples.* Consequently, the health of AIANs is mediated by and construed within a broad historical consciousness of colonial subjugation, and the accompanying bereavement, anomie, indignation, and resistance that has resulted.

The challenge for those dedicated to advancing a culture of health and achieving health equity for AIANs is at least twofold. First, stakeholders must acknowledge upstream determinants of contemporary Indigenous health inequities that research to date has not, and perhaps cannot trace using positivist, Eurocentric research approaches from historical actions, events, policies, and practices to current community health profiles. *That is, the standard of evidence for linking historical oppression and contemporary health inequity must be reconceived and Indigenized.* Second, stakeholders must reframe their thinking and retrain their focus to consider the origins, experiences, attributes, and accounts of Indigenous resurgence in the face of longstanding and overwhelming adversity. *That is, the body of knowledge concerning the health status of Indigenous Americans must shift away from pathology to promise through explorations of resilience, resistance, and well-being.* In this chapter, we explain Indigenous citizenship in Tribal Nations and describe how colonial subjugation impacts health for Indigenous Peoples through settler colonial policies, narratives of pathology, and structural racism and discrimination. After briefly describing the health impacts of colonial subjugation experienced by AIANs, we introduce Indigenous approaches to health which differ from allopathic norms. Finally, we describe the impact of narrative shifting from pathology to promise and the importance of Indigenous governance in research before providing recommendations for addressing health inequity for AIAN Peoples.

Indigenous Citizenship in Tribal Nations

The First Peoples of the lands currently held by the US hail from an array of distinct cultural, political, and racial backgrounds that shape patterns of health and inequity. Given the unique historical, political, and social factors that have impacted Indigenous Peoples since European contact, we have necessarily constrained the focus of this chapter to AIANs, even while strongly affirming that the shared and disparate experiences of our Indigenous relatives not included in this designation, including Latinx Indigenous Peoples, Native Hawaiians, and Pacific Islanders, among others, are equally deserving of scholarly attention.

Millions of Indigenous Peoples inhabited North America prior to contact with Europeans. They created vibrant societies and systems of government that included sophisticated diplomatic practices, justice, health care, and resource management. Most history books, however, frame the roots of the Americas in alignment with European conquest. The tribal sovereignty enjoyed by AIAN Peoples predates the formation of what we know as the United States.[1] Recognized by colonial powers such as the British, Spanish, and French governments through the ratification and enforcement of international treaties, Tribal Nations have a unique sovereign status recognized by the US government.[2]

Upon the formation of the US, the new government included confirmation of the government-to-government relationship with tribes in the US Constitution, within the Commerce Clause, which allows Congress to ratify treaties with Tribal Nations.[3] A basic understanding of this political context is critical. *AIANs share a complex, unique, and constitutionally established relationship with the US government that ensures inherent rights not derived from race or ethnicity.*[1] Federal law and policy distinguish between Indigenous and non-Indigenous peoples. Fundamentally, AIANs are members of sovereign nations, not simply racialized minorities.[4] Therefore, tribes, states, and the federal government comprise three sovereign governing body types under US law.

Colonial Subjugation

Despite the status of AIAN Peoples as citizens of sovereign nations, there is the reality of living in a society in which pseudo-biological notions of race—often determined via arbitrary phenotypic indicators—differentially constrain opportunity. While AIANs are not a race, as a population we are *racialized by the Euro-American majority*, and experience racism and discrimination that have significant deleterious impacts on well-being. Historically, settler populations used racialized language and prejudice in order to "other" AIANs, easing the way for atrocities which enabled westward expansion.[5,6] Later federal policies used racially discriminatory actions to either maintain separation between Indigenous and non-Indigenous populations or force AIANs to assimilate into the mainstream US population. Today, AIANs are over-represented in the federal justice and foster care systems and under-represented in higher education.[7-9] Thus, despite "AIAN" being a socio-political rather than a racial categorization, it is not possible to delve into issues of AIAN health inequity without considering the impacts of structural racism.

There has been a recent move to classify settler colonialism and associated colonial subjugation as social determinants of health for Indigenous Peoples in the Americas.[10,11] While certainly theoretically accurate, terminology such as colonial subjugation is an abstraction that, when used without context, can obfuscate the intent behind and direct relationship between federal Indian policies and deleterious health outcomes. Focusing on colonial harms in the abstract renders the context in which Indigenous health inequity arises invisible, allowing a continuation of the status quo systems and associated federal policies that were explicitly designed for the assimilation and eradication of AIAN Peoples. Such approaches encourage top-down health interventions developed by those outside of communities that pathologize both individuals and entire populations. The focus thus settles on addressing the perceived behavioral inadequacies of Indigenous Peoples (itself a colonial practice) rather than disrupting the systems that function to limit opportunity and maintain structural inequity.[5] In the next section, we introduce some of the policies and practices, from the establishment of the United States to the present, which constitute colonialism and demonstrate the ways in which the subjugation of Indigenous Americans is perpetuated.

Settler Colonial Policies

Impacts of colonization on Indigenous well-being occurred and occur through at least three simultaneous processes: 1) the introduction of disease, both intentionally and unintentionally, by settlers, 2) violent dispossession and erasure through policy (with profound physical, cultural, and spiritual harms), and 3) environmental degradation.[12] Each of these processes is rooted in colonial subjugation. The impact of colonizing forces and the dispossession of tribal lands had sweeping impacts on all tribes across North America. Today, public health practitioners often characterize the impacts of these processes in terms of historical trauma and epistemicide. The term historical trauma refers to the "cumulative emotional and psychological wounding across multiple generations . . . which emanates from massively traumatized group history."[13] Within the AIAN context, historical trauma events are typically widespread within the community, impacting many people, and provoke significant collective distress and mourning.[14] Epistemicide, a related idea, involves the destruction of knowledge, undertaken as a tool of colonization, which has widespread implications for Indigenous well-being.[12]

Research continues to document mental and physical health impacts associated with historical trauma events, called historical trauma responses. These include anxiety, depression, post-traumatic stress disorder (PTSD), substance misuse and substance use disorders, suicidal ideation, and elevated incidence of chronic disease and allostatic load.[15–17] Researchers have documented associations between historical trauma and health in terms of historical cultural losses and psychological distress,[18] residential school experiences and suicidality among First Nations populations in Canada,[19,20] and intergenerational impacts of relocation and residential school policies on parenting, depressive symptoms, and delinquency across generations.[13,21–23] Importantly, experiences of historical trauma may contribute to, interact with, or amplify contemporary trauma experiences and exacerbate negative health outcomes.[23–25]

As a settler colonial state, the overarching goal of the government has, since 1776, been to secure Indigenous lands for settler expansion. Federal policies toward Indigenous Peoples in the Americas are settler–colonial policies. Settler colonialism is an ongoing structure of domination[26] that continues to impact the daily lives of all Americans, Indigenous and otherwise, which differs from classic colonialism in that its aim is land-based, and centers on the acquisition of land in order to enable permanent settlement by colonists.[27] Each phase of US federal Indian policy is directly associated with reducing the rights and access to land for Indigenous peoples, in order to further enable encroachment by settlers, and each is associated with significant historical trauma events. A thorough review of each era is outside of the scope of this chapter. Instead, we introduce a few key laws and policies and their impacts on AIAN health.

The Doctrine of Discovery

Since contact, European settlers acted in accordance with the international law of the Doctrine of Discovery, which justified settler property rights over newly discovered lands and the Indigenous people who lived there. This self-serving law enabled the legal—according to European courts—colonization and settlement of new territories based on presumed superiority over non-European cultures, religions, and people.[28] The Doctrine of Discovery remains international law to this day and was most recently used in 2005 by Justice Ruth Bader Ginsberg in a ruling against the Oneida Nation.[29] The Doctrine of Discovery served as the impetus for each of the policies discussed below, as well as the resulting physical and cultural genocide.

Removal Policies

The Removal Period is defined by the forced removal of Eastern tribes to lands west of the Mississippi and was codified into law by the 1830 Indian Removal Act. The act disregarded hundreds of treaties signed between the federal government and sovereign Tribal Nations, and led to the displacement of more than 46,000 American Indians from their homes and lands between 1830 and 1840,[30,31] including the Cherokee Trail of Tears.[32] In addition to the acute trauma and mortality that resulted immediately from forced removal, the loss of place-based knowledge and connection had severe ramifications for health and spirituality.

Reservation Policies

Starting in the 1850s, the US began to consolidate American Indians west of the Mississippi onto fixed reservations either through direct removal from their traditional lands or through restriction to small holdings. Such segregation further opened territory for settler expansion, while outlawing Indigenous populations from engaging in their traditional life ways.[6] Reservation holdings most frequently represented land poor in resources and challenged Indigenous Peoples' ability to practice traditional means of hunting, fishing, agriculture, and gathering in unfamiliar environments. Removal to reservations also separated Indigenous people from culturally significant and ceremonial sites.[30] As a means of addressing food shortages resulting from relocation and the decimation of major food sources, such as the millions of bison that hundreds of tribes relied upon, the federal government began providing commodity foods to reservations. "Comods," as they came to be known, were high in starch and fat, as compared to the low-fat, antioxidant-rich, protein-dense bison and other wild game, fish, and agricultural products and gathered fruit and vegetables in traditional diets, but provided little in the way of nutritional content.[33,34] Throughout the removal and reservation periods, federal Indian policy fostered Indigenous dependence on the federal government, while maintaining clear separation between Indigenous and settler populations.[32] Reservation policies have been directly associated with elevated rates of chronic disease such as diabetes and cardiovascular disease among AIANs.[33]

Federal Indian Boarding Schools

The Assimilation Era introduced many policies aimed at altering the traditions, cultures, and practices of AIANs in order to more closely align and eventually assimilate AIANs as "productive" members of the dominant Euro-American culture. The kidnapping and forced removal of AIAN children to industrial boarding schools, where they were forced to abandon their culture, traditions, and language and were indoctrinated into Christianity, have been implicated as especially deleterious on mental and physical health across generations. The health impacts of the boarding schools have been widely studied, with results indicating intergenerational impacts on both mental and physical health,[16,17,21,35] aside from the untold number of AIAN children who died or were never able to find their way home.

Allotment

To further federal goals of American Indian assimilation, allotment policies were enacted in 1887. Allotment redefined reservation lands as belonging to individuals, instead of sovereign nations. These lands could then be inherited or sold in keeping with Euro-colonial models of capitalism and paternalism, resulting in reservation lands being further dispossessed by settlers.[32] Allotment did not ensure for family members lands adjacent to one another, resulting in fracturing of family groups and the further interruption of community cohesion.[36] Overall, the assimilation and allotment period is recognized as contributing to deep impoverishment and ethnocide.[37]

Termination

During the Termination Period, spanning the 1940s to the 1980s, the US government sought to limit the number of Tribal Nations to which it had treaty obligations by retracting federal recognition in accordance with a newly developed list of requirements.[30] Ultimately, the termination period resulted in the loss of federal recognition for more than 100 tribes.[30] AIAN identity and tribal citizenship have important implications for health and well-being. Enrolled citizens of federally recognized Tribal Nations have treaty-obligated rights to health care, funded or provided through the federal Indian Health Service. The ability of tribes to invest in services for tribal members such as health care, healthful foods, education, and financial contributions represents an investment in upstream social determinants that are widely recognized to positively impact health outcomes. There has also been significant attention within both the academic literature and popular culture to Indigenous identity politics, particularly as an increasing number of AIANs identify as multi-racial. In addition to the social trends related to AIAN identity both within and outside of AIAN communities, research has shown that multi-racial AIANs and disenrolled AIANs are more likely to report substance use, and are at greater risk of developing suicidal ideation,[38,39] underscoring the need to better understand the connection between identity, sense of belonging, and health, as well as calling attention to the need for further research into the devastating and ongoing effects of the Termination Era.

Relocation

Concurrent with termination, the federal government also initiated active policies focused on the relocation of AIANs away from reservations and into urban centers. Cities were advertised as providing opportunities for education, training, and employment. Relocating AIANs from reservations to cities supported the government's desire to divest from responsibilities to Tribal Nations.[30,40] While financial and educational opportunities were more plentiful in cities, the federal Bureau of Indian Affairs failed to predict the challenges of acculturation for a population previously kept largely segregated, and racism emerged as a significant barrier to accessing housing and other community resources for recent migrants. Additionally, as people with strong ties to community and kinship networks, the reality of urban life, in which AIANs represented only a tiny fraction of the population, led many to experience significant isolation.[30] Today, AIAN people make up a large proportion of the unhoused population in many urban centers.[41]

Narratives of Pathology

Formal colonial policies were aided by informal, but no less damaging, practices that served to "other," oppress, and/or erase AIAN peoples in the eyes of the settler majority. While the methods have changed over time, the harms inflicted upon AIANs remain very real.

Historical Context

Deficit-focused narratives and negative stereotypes for Indigenous Peoples can be linked to European invasion. As Europeans traveled back and forth between the Americas and Europe, they used printing presses to report their experiences.[42] These reports document early negative stereotypes, such as Indigenous Peoples as "treacherous savages," that continue to persist today.[42] Indeed, the US Declaration of Independence refers to the First Peoples of the land as "merciless Indian Savages."[43] Such dehumanization of Indigenous Peoples was used to justify settler land theft and genocide via federal policies. For example, many of the federal policies introduced previously were implemented to "civilize" AIANs and to solve the "Indian problem."[44]

Contemporary Context

Inaccurate stereotypes about AIANs continue to pervade US society.[45] Stereotypes about AIANs as uncivilized, primitive, uneducated, and one homogeneous group perpetuate racism and are transmitted via textbooks, movies and TV shows, commercial logos, tourist attraction imagery, sports teams, and academic publications.[45,46] AIANs also face another form of discrimination: invisibility.[47] Invisibility creates harm in that non-AIANs then create their own narratives about AIANs, including negative stereotypes perpetuated in media.[47]

Negative narratives and stereotypes have detrimental impacts on the provision of healthcare services, on AIAN health, and on health research. The dominance of a Western biomedical model leads to the pathologization and problematization of individual health,[48] rather than a critique of the systems and histories from which contemporary health inequities stem. *The normalized perception of Indigenous Peoples and communities as unhealthy is rooted in colonialist propaganda and is maintained by top-down, extractive public health research and practice that benefits individual health researchers and settler institutions while actively harming or passively neglecting Indigenous Peoples.*

Mounting research demonstrates the harms associated with negative stereotypes of AIANs, including impacts to self-esteem and psychological well-being.[46] Further, ongoing discrimination informs policy by threatening the protection of sovereignty and treaty rights. Rather than celebrating Indigenous strengths and diversity of culture, such discrimination undermines the fundamental humanity and dignity of AIANs.[47]

Structural Racism and Discrimination

Through this introduction to federal Indian policy and associated narratives of pathology we demonstrate that, while it is true that many commonly recognized social determinants of ill health have adversely impacted the well-being of AIANs, the roots of this legacy of disadvantage are found in centuries of settler-colonial policies and actions with their basis in White supremacy. *Consequently, the health of Indigenous Peoples is mediated by and construed within a broad historical consciousness of colonial subjugation, and the accompanying bereavement, anomie, indignation, and resistance that has resulted.*

The impacts of policy are compounded by contemporary racism and discrimination, which have long been demonstrated to affect health at the individual and community level in non-AIAN communities.[49,50] Both in adolescence and adulthood, there is evidence, drawn from AIANs as well

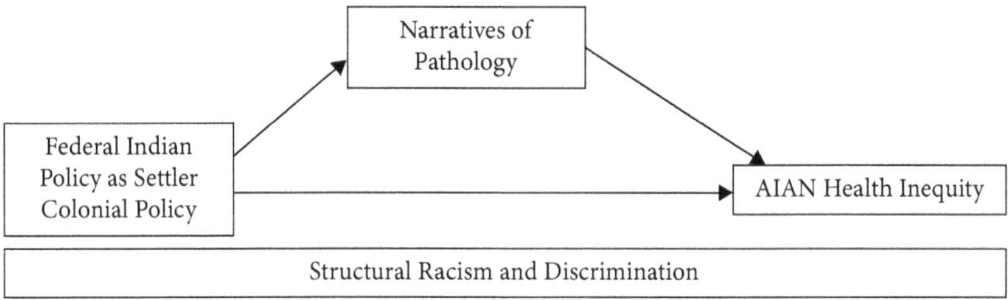

Figure 7.1 Conceptual model of colonial subjugation and Indigenous health inequity

as other minoritized populations in the US, that perceived discrimination can act as a psychological stressor, contributing to lower self-esteem, depression, and psychological distress.[51–54] Indeed, research (Figure 7.1) has found an association between family histories of historical trauma and greater vulnerability to perceived discrimination, including in healthcare settings,[55,56] as an ongoing traumatic stressor.[14,57,58]

Further, demonstrated AIAN inequities across multiple social determinants of health implicate structural racism as continuing to impact AIANs at the individual, family, and community level.[14,59] Thus, federal Indian policies—as settler colonial policies—have adversely impacted AIAN health status directly through violent dispossession, and indirectly through intentional othering and the resulting narratives of pathology, structural racism, and discrimination.

Tracing the causal chain from Euro-American colonial subjugation to Indigenous community health inequities is challenging, due in part to methodological complications of linking 500 years of settler colonial policies to present-day health problems in the context of the great diversity of people and experiences throughout "Indian Country." Nevertheless, there can be no doubt that Indigenous health and well-being exhibited a precipitous decline in the wake of colonial dispossession and subjugation.

A public health emphasis on the social determinants of health would typically attribute striking Indigenous health inequities to poverty, demoralization, and despair. Certainly, a decline in health and well-being would be expected for peoples weathering circumstances of extreme deprivation, communal disruption, or societal collapse. But for Indigenous Americans, these deprivations and disruptions in most instances were deliberately engineered by others.

Specifically, *Indigenous disadvantage has resulted from long efforts to intentionally dispossess, contain, control, marginalize, and erase, even via extermination.* Thus, Indigenous community health inequities are the contemporary "downstream" indicators of barbaric historical projects of colonization.[60–62] Efforts by the federal government to begin addressing the root causes of Indigenous dis-ease in the US have been limited, with even a formal apology still outstanding.

Health Impacts of Colonial Subjugation

Prior to colonization, Indigenous Peoples were healthy and living according to cultural values, worldviews, and traditions with land-based knowledges.[63] Following European contact, settler-colonial policies and ongoing interpersonal and structural racism led to a health crisis for Indigenous populations.[64] There is evidence that several health inequities observed among AIANs today are relatively recent in history, and many contemporary health inequities can be attributed to the lasting impacts of contact, colonization, and oppression.

Such health inequity is most readily apparent when comparing average life expectancy: in 2019, AIANs broadly could expect, at birth, to live 78.4 years, while the expected age for White Americans at the same time was 80.6. The causes of this discrepancy were exacerbated by the COVID-19 pandemic, with life expectancy for AIANs during this time dropping more than six years.[65] In addition to lower life expectancy, AIANs experience disproportionately high rates of exposure to Adverse Childhood Experiences and affiliated worse health outcomes,[15] poorer mental health,[66,67] elevated rates of substance misuse and disorders,[16,67,68] suicidality,[69,70] and chronic and acute diseases including type 2 diabetes,[71] cardiovascular disease,[72] cancers,[73] tuberculosis,[74] influenza,[75] and sexually transmitted infections.[74] While statistics differ by Tribal Nation, the overwhelming pattern is one of extreme inequity in both mental and physical health between AIANs and other racialized populations in the United States.

It is important to recognize, however, that these statistics capture only a small segment of a biased portrayal and likely do so inaccurately. This is not to deny that striking inequities exist, but rather (as we detail in this chapter) that AIAN perceptions of health, well-being, and success are not synonymous with Euro-centric definitions, and that significant error exists in research undertaken with Indigenous Peoples in the US. It is also important to note that, while health disparities are a very real concern for AIAN communities, we are not defined by narratives of poor health. Therefore, in this chapter, we adhere to what Aleut scholar Eve Tuck calls desire-based rather than damage-centered perspectives of Indigenous health,[76] namely, that which engages the complexity, self-determination, and strength of Indigenous Peoples rather than framing entire communities as unidimensional, depleted, and damaged.[76] Thus, we actively and intentionally highlight the historical, structural, and systemic causes of health inequity. Moreover, we emphasize the ways that AIAN worldviews and approaches to well-being, as well as an intentional re-framing of narratives from pathology to promise, can interrupt these processes of dis-ease.

Indigenous Approaches to Health

As we imagine a future marked by Indigenous health equity, transformation cannot be achieved without the inclusion of Indigenous culture, knowledge, worldviews, current wellness practices, and traditional systems of health. The preservation and practice of pre-colonial wellness traditions have been the foundation of survival for AIANs while navigating genocide; dispossession of land, knowledge, and culture; perpetual assaults on our lifeways and health; and the present-day health disparities and inequities that have resulted. Importantly, Indigenous worldviews and practices prioritize the maintenance of balance among all humans, other living beings, and the land.

There are as many Indigenous concepts and practices of wellness as there are tribal communities. Therefore, we cannot assume the generalizability of any successful Indigenous health program or health system. We can, however, continue to support the revitalization of Indigenous health traditions and systems, financially and politically, within every Indigenous community. This support is especially imperative considering the trust responsibility that the US maintains with each individual sovereign Tribal Nation. Implementation and development of integrative and culturally derived approaches to health and well-being must be guided by the following core commitments that emerged from a recent Indigenous Traditional Medicine Summit: Perception (a framing of Indigenous health as entailing Spirituality), Translation (an explanation of Indigenous healing practices for a broader audience with attending Humility), Protection (a concern for preserving long-endangered Indigenous healing practices with an eye toward Sustainability), and Contribution (a desire to partner with outsiders in the promotion of Indigenous healing so long as there is Accountability).[77]

Broadly, Indigenous concepts of health and wellness differ from biomedical concepts, and Indigenous well-being cannot be fully achieved through Euro-colonial frameworks. It is essential that entities supporting Indigenous well-being fundamentally shift expectations into alignment with Indigenous frameworks and worldviews, which may differ dramatically in terms of measurement and outcome assessment. The key concepts of well-being described below are central to effective health systems for Indigenous Peoples. The vision of health equity must weave Indigenous concepts and worldviews into existing health delivery systems to be effective. Environments of inclusion will normalize Indigenous culture, Traditional Medicine practitioners, and identified healers. Health systems must also discern levels of cultural safety, appropriateness, sensitivity, and alignment, which necessitates the inclusion of compensated Indigenous cultural experts to assist with discerning cultural safety in the process. Environments of inclusion will create spaces for health and well-being.

Traditional Practices of Wellness

Traditional Indigenous ways of life are still practiced today at various levels of maintenance and revitalization. These life ways consist of speaking one's Indigenous language, engaging in traditional spiritual practices, participating in community events, harvesting, preparing and sharing traditional foods, knowing ancestral genealogies, and following traditional forms of politics and leadership (e.g., eliciting knowledge and guidance from Elders, adhering to clan roles). *Engaging with each aspect of these traditional life ways is associated with positive health outcomes including greater mental well-being, reduced substance misuse, and greater physical wellness.*[78,79] In addition, Indigenous Peoples have health-specific resources, which include healing ceremonies, trained health practitioners, and traditional medicines.

Indigenous People have unique worldviews and perspectives, which derive most notably from Indigenous languages and spirituality. Worldviews shape decision making, problem solving, and idea generation, while the construction of worldviews promoted through colonialism suppresses political and social growth.[80] Indigenous worldviews vary but often center the reciprocal relationships embedded within broader fields of connectedness with respect to spiritual, environmental, and intergenerational domains.[90,98]

Reciprocal Relationships

Relationships between the individual, family, community, ancestors, nature, and spirits must be nourished for Indigenous Peoples to achieve wellness. Indigenous models of health often center the individual within the greater relational framework.[81–83] Language and cultural engagement deepen relationships with spiritual helpers, community members, and with the earth.[79] It is believed that when individuals, within each of their roles as heads of households, community leaders, youth, or Elders begin to "live well," the health of those existing within the surrounding relational networks will begin to approach wellness.

Connectedness

Indigenous spirituality is at the center of many models of Indigenous well-being.[81,84,85] Spirituality is comprised of mindset, worldview, and individual and community rituals and practices that collectively shape, guide, and connect individuals to beliefs, values, higher powers, and purpose. Research has shown an association between higher levels of spirituality and reduced suicidal thoughts[86] and substance use,[87,88] and improved mental health.[89] Spiritual health is linked to physical, mental, and emotional health, and, for Indigenous Peoples, cannot be separated from these other domains of well-being.[90]

Relationships with the land are critical aspects of wellness for Indigenous Peoples, including harmony with all living beings,[85] environmental connectedness,[81] narrative connection with the land,[84] and land as a living member of the family.[83] Since time immemorial, the land has contributed to health by providing the sustenance resources necessary for survival (i.e., nutrition, medicine, clothes, shelter); being a physical and spiritual medium for spiritual connection, environmental connection, and worldview; and providing the space for community cohesion, connectedness, and belonging.[91]

Connecting to ancestors, history, culture, and health via the land is applied by various programs aimed to revitalize cultural forms of healing and strength.[92,93]

Positive effects of living on one's ancestral homelands and engaging in land-based cultural activities have been associated with self-reported happiness,[94] and a 2021 systematic review found 28 published academic papers that supported that land, sea, and subsistence-based living were important to Indigenous well-being.[90] Reconnecting to our traditional foods by hunting, fishing, and gathering, and using values of reciprocity (e.g., taking only what you need and allowing regeneration), we can affect the balance of the ecosystem in a positive way, creating sources of sustenance and health for generations to come.

When we practice our Indigenous ways of life, we are connected to our spiritual helpers, to our broader community, and to an intergenerational continuum that spans from our ancestors to future generations.[81,95] Many Indigenous Peoples in the US recognize a Seventh Generation Prophecy that encourages behaviors that ensure the preservation of the same cultural and environmental gifts that we are afforded today for our descendants, seven generations into the future. In this way, we are connected to our ancestors and have inherited this responsibility for future generations. Indigenous wellness is guided by this interconnectivity of past, present, and future, and the practices and worldviews that protect it.

Narrative Shifting from Pathology to Promise

There is an active movement to shift narratives about Indigenous Peoples away from pathology and toward promise. Language matters and helps shift narratives away from deficit, pathology, and problems, and toward strengths and resilience. Native "survivance"—a portmanteau of survival and resistance—denotes an ongoing presence and vital persistence of AIANs instead of historical erasure and victim-based narratives.[96] Advances have been made through a national Indigenous-led non-profit "IllumiNative," whose mission is to increase AIAN visibility and challenge negative narratives about AIANs throughout the US.[97] Other impactful projects are being led by Indigenous researchers. "OrigiNatives" is an Indigenous-led digital storytelling project that aims to shift power to AIANs themselves rather than perpetuating harmful colonial narratives about what it means to be AIAN.[98] *Broadcasting Indigenous voices of strength is an essential tool to counter the dominance of historically traumatic experiences of Indigenous Peoples.* This approach also complements the work of strategic AIAN-led efforts to center community assets and counter dominant headlines and narratives that create dismay and reinforce damaging stereotypes about Indigenous Peoples.[99] It is essential to support Indigenous leadership as a means of advancing mainstream narratives of Indigenous strength and promise, including in health care and research fields. There is a growing call to advance strengths-based approaches to Indigenous health research from Indigenous leaders, scholars, and practitioners asking for research to build upon existing community strengths and well-being.[100] Alongside their communities, Indigenous scholars are leading the development of new frameworks that highlight Indigenous epistemologies and traditions and advance scientific research.[81,101]

Indigenous Governance in Research

Indigenous communities have conducted research since time immemorial to relate with the environment for the benefit of people, animals, and the natural world. Indigenous protocols of knowledge development and knowledge transmission are carefully intertwined with land-based practices, spiritual connectedness, and Elder leadership. Settler colonialism has sought and continues to suppress and ignore Indigenous research methodologies and methods.[102] Increasingly, *Indigenous Peoples, particularly in the US, are engaging with research, asserting oversight of research and data obtained on tribal lands (or with their citizens), and exercising authority over research that affects their interests.*

Community/Tribally-Based Participatory Research

Community-based participatory research (CBPR) has become a standard research practice for academics and minoritized communities to address complex health issues.[103,104] The CBPR research paradigm fully engages and partners with members of the communities that the research aims to serve.[105] Tribally based participatory research (TBPR) is a subset of CBPR developed specifically for research with Tribal Nations.[106,107] While much of the CBPR literature is focused on work with racialized populations, TBPR explicitly focuses on research between sovereign entities, as AIANs are citizens of sovereign nations as opposed to another racialized group. These processes require additional formal resolutions, training requirements, and presentations to engage tribal government-level stakeholders. The TBPR paradigm also necessitates a deeper understanding of cultural norms and protocols, and the employment of community members on the research team.[108]

Tribal Oversight in Research

Tribal Nations rely on a number of mechanisms to review, approve, manage, and control research within their jurisdictions and beyond. Some tribes have their own policies and procedures for research oversight (e.g., tribal research review boards). Other tribes use tribal colleges, tribal organizations, or the Indian Health Service to conduct research oversight for them.[109] Today, tribes also use tribal codes and resolutions to define their expectations for jurisdiction over research and data.[110,111]

Previous and current data collection, storage, and use may not align with Indigenous communities' rights, responsibilities, and interests. Often, such research practices fail to benefit the communities from which the data arise and result in biases in analysis and use of the data.[112] As health research and data advance within open science and big data contexts, the potential for bias and harm to further negatively impact Indigenous communities grows. Indigenous Peoples have responded to these challenges by asserting rights and responsibilities to human and non-human kin through research oversight and data governance practices.[112–117]

Institutional Inclusion of Indigenous People

To increase equity in Indigenous well-being, it is essential to increase equity in research. Toward this end, it is critical that institutions recruit, retain, and promote Indigenous Peoples and associated research methodologies. The former comprises Indigenous researchers, as well as Indigenous community experts. *To advance self-determination among Indigenous Peoples, institutions must recognize that Indigenous health research is occurring outside of universities and research centers, and within Indigenous communities where Indigenous Peoples are active leaders in developing research agendas.*

According to the National Science Foundation, AIANs consistently earn fewer than 1 percent of doctorates awarded in science and engineering, hampering the extent to which Indigenous researchers can be included in institutions. Indeed, AIANs are appointed to the rank of full professor in only 6 of fifteen of the nation's top STEM departments.[118] Thus, it is crucial that institutions establish mechanisms for supporting and including Indigenous Peoples and associated methodologies in an equitable manner, including research policy, funding structures, and other strategic efforts.

Closing Recommendations for Addressing AIAN Health Inequity

Addressing health inequities experienced by AIANs must occur through: 1) recognizing and grappling with the legacy of colonial subjugation, enacted through policies, narratives of pathology, and structural racism, 2) embracing Indigenous strengths and perceptions of health as valid and viable means of health promotion, and 3) interrupting entrenched hierarchies such that Indigenous sovereignty is upheld and Indigenous leadership is prioritized at every stage of research. Toward this aim, we offer three recommendations for policymakers, health researchers, and advocacy groups.

First, it is essential to understand that Indigenous perceptions of health and wellness differ from the biomedical understandings prioritized by the Euro-colonial majority. In order to address AIAN health inequity, health research and interventions must intentionally dismantle existing ideas around health and healing and re-align them with Indigenous concepts, traditions, and practices of health.

Second, existing hierarchies must intentionally dismantle research gate-keeping by funders and oversight bodies (e.g., Institutional Review Boards). Such bodies have traditionally functioned as barriers for Indigenous health research and interventions based in and accountable to AIAN communities. In order to improve Indigenous health equity, it is necessary that research that is conducted *by* and *with* Tribal Nations be prioritized over research conducted *on* Indigenous communities and bodies without community input. This research must be strengths-based (or "desire-based") and unequivocally acknowledge colonization and structural racism as the fundamental causes of health inequities experienced by AIANs and of dis-ease and dis-order among all Americans. In order to ensure equity, all research involving AIAN participants must include a descriptive statement concerning Indigenous authorship and collaboration, and should also include collaboration statements from tribal partners. Furthermore, all research that includes AIAN participants should include a data sovereignty statement that ensures data and materials protections. These should be developed in collaboration with, or by, each Tribal Nation whose members are included in the research, recognizing that each community has different priorities and concerns.

Finally, there must be investment in tribally controlled research capacity. At the personnel level, it is essential that research and funding institutions support the growing network of Indigenous researchers through both funding streams as well as education and mentorship opportunities. For this to be effective, institutes of higher education must be re-structured to be welcoming and supportive environments for students holding minoritized identities, including Indigenous students. These efforts must be inclusive of students enrolled in Tribal Colleges and Universities. By fostering the development of Indigenous researchers, we not only build tribal capacity and ability to conduct community-driven research, we invest in the development of evidence-based health research and interventions stemming from Indigenous ways of knowing and being as well as perceptions of wellness. Similarly, supporting Indigenous researchers increases the likelihood that structural and historical health determinants will be appropriately investigated as contributing to health inequity and that culturally appropriate tests and measures are developed and used to assess the health of Indigenous Peoples. Building research infrastructure within Tribal Nations will also work to destabilize entrenched power hierarchies within which academic researchers and institutions are at the top and Indigenous Peoples are at the bottom. This restructuring will pave the way for mainstream funders to confidently award research grants directly to AIAN communities.

Acknowledgements

The author team wishes to thank Fiona Grubin for her contributions to this work as Project Coordinator, and Delaney Ignace, Skylar Smith, and Lena Tinker for their contributions as undergraduate Research Assistants. The authors have no conflicts of interest to report.

References

1. National Congress of American Indians. *Tribal Nations and the United States: An introduction.* 2020:11. https://archive.ncai.org/about-tribes.
2. Getches D, Wilkinson C, Williams R, Fletcher M, Carpenter K. *Cases and materials on Federal Indian law.* 7th ed. St Paul, MN: West Academic Publishing; 2017.
3. US Constitution, Article 1, Section 8, Clause 3.
4. Wilkins DE, Kiiwetinepinesiik Stark H. *American Indian politics and the American political system.* 4th ed. Lanham, MD: Rowman & Littlefield; 2018.
5. Smith LT. *Decolonizing methodologies: Research and Indigenous peoples.* 3rd ed. London: Bloomsbury Academic; 2021.
6. Dunbar-Ortiz R. *An Indigenous Peoples' history of the United States.* Boston, MA: Beacon Press; 2014.
7. National Indian Child Welfare Association. *Time for reform: A matter of justice for American Indian and Alaska Native children.* The PEW Charitable Trust; 2007.
8. Cunneen C, Tauri JM. Indigenous Peoples, criminology, and criminal justice. *Annual Review of Criminology.* 2019;2(1):359–381. doi:10.1146/annurev-criminol-011518-024630
9. Brayboy BMJ, Solyom JA, Castagno AE. Indigenous Peoples in higher education. *Journal of American Indian Education.* 2015;54(1):154–186.
10. Czyzewski K. Colonialism as a broader social determinant of health. *iipj.* 2011;2(1). doi:10.18584/iipj.2011.2.1.5
11. Kim PJ. Social determinants of health inequities in Indigenous Canadians through a life course approach to colonialism and the Residential School system. *Health Equity.* 2019;3(1):378–381. doi:10.1089/heq.2019.0041
12. Hall BL, Tandon R. Decolonization of knowledge, epistemicide, participatory research and higher education. *Research for All.* 2017;1(1):6–19.
13. Brave Heart MYH. The historical trauma response among Natives and its relationship with substance abuse: A Lakota illustration. *Journal of Psychoactive Drugs.* 2003;35(1): 7–13. doi:10.1080/02791072.2003.10399988
14. Evans-Campbell T. Historical trauma in American Indian/Native Alaska Communities: A multilevel framework for exploring impacts on individuals, families, and communities. *Journal of Interpersonal Violence.* 2008;23(3):316–338. doi:10.1177/08862605073 12290
15. Moon-Riley KC, Copeland JL, Metz GA, Currie CL. The biological impacts of parental residential school attendance on the next generation. *SSM—Population Health.* 2018:100343. doi:10.1016/j.ssmph.2018.100343
16. Gone JP, Hartmann WE, Pomerville A, Wendt DC, Klem SH, Burrage RL. The impact of historical trauma on health outcomes for Indigenous populations in the USA and Canada: A systematic review. *American Psychologist.* 2019;74(1):20–35.
17. Running Bear U, Thayer ZM, Croy CD, Kaufman CE, Manson SM. The impact of individual and parental American Indian boarding school attendance on chronic physical health of Northern Plains tribes: *Family & Community Health.* 2019;42(1):1–7. doi:10.1097/FCH.0000000000000205
18. Whitbeck LB, Walls, ML, Johnson KD, Morrisseau AD, McDougall CM. Depressed affect and historical loss among North American Indigenous adolescents. *AIANMHR.* 2009;16(3):16–41. doi:10.5820/aian.1603.2009.16
19. Elias B, Mignone J, Hall M, Hong SP, Hart L, Sareen J. Trauma and suicide behaviour histories among a Canadian indigenous population: An empirical exploration of the potential role of Canada's residential school system. *Social Science & Medicine.* 2012;74(10):1560–1569. doi:10.1016/j.socscimed.2012.01.026

20. Wilk P, Maltby A, Cooke M. Residential schools and the effects on Indigenous health and well-being in Canada-a scoping review. *Public Health Review*. 2017;38:8. doi:10.1186/s40985-017-0055-6

21. Bombay A, Matheson K, Anisman H. The intergenerational effects of Indian Residential Schools: Implications for the concept of historical trauma. *Transcultural Psychiatry*. 2014;51(3):320–338. doi:10.1177/1363461513503380

22. Bombay A, Matheson K, Anisman H. The impact of stressors on second generation Indian residential school survivors. *Transcultural Psychiatry*. 2011;48(4):367–391. doi:10.1177/1363461511410240

23. Walls ML, Whitbeck LB. Advantages of stress process approaches for measuring historical trauma. *The American Journal of Drug and Alcohol Abuse*. 2012;38(5):416–420. doi:10.3109/00952990.2012.694524

24. Brockie T, Heinzelmann M, Gill J. A framework to examine the role of epigenetics in health disparities among Native Americans. *Nursing Research and Practice*. Published online December 9, 2013:1–9. doi:10.1155/2013/410395

25. Gillson SL, Hautala D, Sittner KJ, Walls M. Historical trauma and oppression: Associations with internalizing outcomes among American Indian adults with type 2 diabetes. *Transcult Psychiatry*. 2022;61(3):1–13. doi:10.1177/13634615221079146

26. Wolfe P. *Settler colonialism and the transformation of anthropology: The politics and poetics of an ethnographic event*. London: Cassell; 1999.

27. Glenn EN. Settler colonialism as structure: A framework for comparative studies of US race and gender formation. *Sociology of Race and Ethnicity*. 2015;1(1):52–72. doi:10.1177/2332649214560440

28. Miller RJ, Ruru J, Behrendt L, Lindberg T. *Discovering Indigenous lands: The doctrine of discovery in the English colonies*. Oxford: Oxford University Press; 2010.

29. Goldberg C. Finding the way to Indian country: Justice Ruth Bader Ginsburg's decisions in Indian law cases. *Ohio State Law Journal*. 2009;70(4):1003–1035.

30. Prucha FP. *The great father: The United States government and the American Indians*. Lincoln, NE: University of Nebraska Press; 1995.

31. Prucha FP. *American Indian policy in crisis: Christian reformers and the Indians*. Norman, OK: University of Oklahoma Press; 1976.

32. Black JE. *American Indians and the rhetoric of removal and allotment*. Jackson, MI: University Press of Mississippi; 2015.

33. Wiedman D. Native American embodiment of the chronicities of modernity: Reservation food, diabetes, and the metabolic syndrome among the Kiowa, Comanche, and Apache. *Medical Anthropology Quarterly*. 2012;26(4):595–612. doi:10.1111/maq.12009

34. Jernigan AK. Embodied heritage: Obesity, cultural identity, and food distribution programs in the Choctaw Nation of Oklahoma. [PhD, University of Massachusetts, Amherst; 2018]. https://scholarworks.umass.edu/server/api/core/bitstreams/b9d756fa-472f-4049-ba52-48efc6d15250/content.

35. Evans-Campbell T, Walters KL, Pearson CR, Campbell CD. Indian boarding school experience, substance use, and mental health among urban two-spirit American Indian/Alaska Natives. *The American Journal of Drug and Alcohol Abuse*. 2012;38(5):421–427. doi:10.3109/00952990.2012.701358

36. Rusco E. The Indian Reorganization Act and Indian self-government. In: Lemont ED, ed. *American Indian constitutional reform and the rebuilding of Native nations*. Austin, TX: University of Texas Press; 2006:49–104. doi:10.7560/712812-005

37. Talbot S. Indian Reorganization Act: 1934. In: Gallagher CA, Lippard CD, eds. *Race and racism in the United States: An encyclopedia of the American mosaic*. Santa Barbara, CA: Greenwood; 2014.

38. Parker M, Duran B, Rhew I, Magarati M, Larimer M, Donovan DM. Risk and protective factors associated with moderate and acute suicidal ideation among a national sample of tribal college and university students. *Journal of Rural Health*. 2021;37(3):545–553.

39. Subica AM, Wu LT. Substance use and suicide in Pacific Islander, American Indian, and multiracial youth. *American Journal of Preventative Medicine*. 2018;54(6):795–805.

40. Miller DK. Willing Workers: Urban Relocation and American Indian Initiative, 1940s–1960s. *Ethnohistory*. 2013;60(1):51–76. doi:10.1215/00141801-1816175

41. Substance Abuse and Mental Health Services Administration. *Expert panel on homelessness among American Indians, Alaska Natives, and Native Hawaiians*. 2012.

42. Calloway CG. *First Peoples: A documentary survey of American Indian history*. 4th ed. Bedford/St. Martins: Macmillan; 2012.

43. *U.S. Declaration of Independence*. 1776.

44. Brave Heart MYH, DeBruyn L. The American Indian holocaust: Healing historical unresolved grief. *American Indian and Alaska Native Mental Health Research*. 1998;8(2): 56–78.

45. Mihesuah DA. *American Indians: Stereotypes & realities*. Atlanta, GA: Clarity; 1996.

46. Davis-Delano LR, Gone JP, Fryberg SA. The psychosocial effects of Native American mascots: A comprehensive review of empirical research findings. *Race, Ethnicity, and Education*. 2020;23(5):613–633.

47. First Nations Development Institute. *Compilation of all research from the Reclaiming Native Truth project*. Published online 2018. http://firstnations.org/publications/compilation-of-all-research-from-the-reclaiming-native-truth-project/.

48. Wexler LM, Gone JP. Culturally responsive suicide prevention in indigenous communities: unexamined assumptions and new possibilities. *American Journal of Public Health*. 2012;102(5):800–806.

49. Williams DR, Mohammed SA. Racism and health I: Pathways and scientific evidence. *American Behavioral Scientist*. 2013;57(8):1152–1173. doi:10.1177/0002764213487340

50. Geronimus AT. The weathering hypothesis and the health of African-American women and infants: Evidence and speculations. *Ethnicity & Disease*. 1992;2(3):207–221.

51. Whitbeck LB. The beginnings of mental health disparities: Emergent mental disorders among Indigenous adolescents. In: Carlo G, Crockett LJ, Carranza MA, eds. *Health Disparities in Youth and Families*. New York: Springer; 2011:121–149. doi:10.1007/978-1-4419-7092-3_6

52. Krieger N, Smith K, Naishadham D, Hartman C, Barbeau EM. Experiences of discrimination: Validity and reliability of a self-report measure for population health research on racism and health. *Social Science & Medicine*. 2005;61(7):1576–1596. doi:10.1016/j.socscimed.2005.03.006

53. Flores E, Tschann JM, Dimas JM, Pasch LA, de Groat CL. Perceived racial/ethnic discrimination, posttraumatic stress symptoms, and health risk behaviors among Mexican American adolescents. *Journal of Counseling Psychology*. 2010;57(3):264–273. doi:10.1037/a0020026

54. Whitbeck LB, Hoyt DR, McMorris BJ, Chen X, Stubben JD. Perceived discrimination and early substance abuse among American Indian children. *Journal of Health and Social Behavior*. 2001;42(4):405. doi:10.2307/3090187

55. Jaramillo ET, Haozous E, Willging CE. The community as the unit of healing: Conceptualizing social determinants of health and well-being for older American Indian adults. *The Gerontologist*. 2022;62(5):732–741. doi:10.1093/geront/gnac018

56. Walls M, Gonzalez J, Gladney T, Onello E. Unconscious biases: Racial microaggressions in American Indian health care. *Journal of the American Board of Family Medicine*. 2015;28(2):231–239.

57. Walters KL, Simoni JM. Reconceptualizing Native women's health: An "Indigenist" stress-coping model. *American Journal of Public Health*. 2002;92(4):520–524. doi:10.2105/AJPH.92.4.520

58. Myhra LL. "It runs in the family": Intergenerational transmission of historical trauma among urban American Indians and Alaska Natives in culturally specific sobriety maintenance programs. *American Indian and Alaska Native Mental Health Research*. 2011;18(2):17–40. doi:10.5820/aian.1802.2011.17

59. Kirmayer LJ, Gone JP, Moses J. Rethinking historical trauma. *Transcultural Psychiatry*. 2014;51(3):299–319.

60. Jones D. The persistence of American Indian health disparities. *The American Journal of Public Health*. 2006;96(12):2122–2134.

61. King M, Smith A, Gracey M. Indigenous health part 2: The underlying causes of the health gap. *The Lancet*. 2009;374(9683):76–85. doi:10.1016/S0140-6736(09)60827-8

62. Warne D, Lajimodiere D. American Indian health disparities: psychosocial influences. *Social and Personality Psychology Compass*. 2015;9(10):567–579.

63. Echo-Hawk A. *Indigenous health equity*. Seattle, WA: Urban Indian Health Institute; 2019.

64. Centers for Disease Control and Prevention. Web-based Injury Statistics Query and Reporting System (WISQARS). Accessed April 21, 2021. https://wisqars.cdc.gov/.

65. Romero S, Caryn Rabin R, Walker M. How the pandemic shortened life expectancy in Indigenous communities: New federal data outline the scale of suffering among Native Americans and Alaska Natives. *New York Times*. August 31, 2022. https://www.nytimes.com/2022/08/31/health/life-expectancy-covid-native-americans-alaskans.html.

66. Gone J, Trimble J. American Indian and Alaska Native mental health: Diverse perspectives on enduring disparities. *Annual Review of Clinical Psychology*. 2012;8:131–160.

67. Brave Heart MYH, Elkins J, Martin J, Mootz J, Chase J, Nanez J. Women finding the way: American Indian women leading intervention research in Native communities. *American Indian and Alaska Native Mental Health Research*. 2016;23(3):24–47.

68. Wendt DC, Hartmann WE, Allen J, et al. Substance use research with Indigenous communities. *American Journal of Community Psychology*. 2019;64(1–2):146–158.

69. Johns Hopkins Center for American Indian Health. *CULTURE FORWARD: A strengths and culture based tool to protect our Native youth from suicide*. Accessed October 17, 2025. https://cih.jhu.edu/programs/cultureforward.

70. Centers for Disease Control and Prevention, National Center for Health Statistics. *1999–2020 Wide Ranging Online Data for Epidemiological Research (WONDER), Multiple Cause of Death Files* [data file]. 2021. Accessed August 12, 2022. http://wonder.cdc.gov/ucd-icd10.html.

71. Office of Minority Health. *Diabetes and American Indians/Alaska Natives*. Washington, DC: US Department of Health and Human Services; 2021.

72. Breathett K, Sims M, Gross M, et al. Cardiovascular health in American Indians and Alaska Natives: A scientific statement from the American Heart Association. *Circulation*. 2020;141(25):e948–e959.

73. Melkonian SC, Weir HK, Jim MA, Preikschat B, Haverkamp D, White MC. Incidence of and trends in the leading cancers with elevated incidence among American Indian and Alaska Native populations, 2012–2016. *American Journal of Epidemiology*. 2020;190(4):528–538.

74. Centers for Disease Control and Prevention. *Health disparities in HIV, viral hepatitis, STDs, and TB: American Indians and Alaska Natives*. Atlanta, GA: Centers for Disease Control and Prevention; 2020.

75. Doxey M, Chrzaszcz L, Dominguez A, James RD. A forgotten danger: Burden of influenza mortality among American Indians and Alaska Natives, 1999–2016. *Journal of Public Health Management and Practice*. 2019;25(5):s7–s10.

76. Tuck E. Suspending damage: A letter to communities. *Harvard Educational Review*. 2009;79(3):409–427.

77. National Institutes of Health. *2019 traditional medicine summit report: Maintaining and protecting culture through healing*. Bethesda, MA: National Institutes of Health; 2019. http://dpcpsi.nih.gov/sites/default/files/NIH-THRO-2019-Traditional-Medicine-Summit-Report.pdf.

78. Carr T, Chartier B, Dadgostari T. "I'm not really healed . . . I'm just bandaged up": Perceptions of healing among former students of Indian residential schools. *International Journal of Indigenous Health*. 2017;12(1):39–56. doi:10.18357/ijih121201716901

79. Beltran R, Schultz K, Fernandez AR, Walters K L, Duran B. From ambivalence to revitalization: Negotiating cardiovascular health behaviors related to environmental and historical trauma in a Northwest American Indian community. *American Indian and Alaska Native Mental Health Research.* 2018;25(2):103–128.

80. Crawford J. Endangered Native American language: what is to be done? *The Bilingual Research Journal.* 1995;19(1):17–38.

81. Ullrich JS. For the love of our children: An Indigenous connectedness framework. *AlterNative: An International Journal of Indigenous Peoples.* 2019;15(2):121–130. doi:10.1177/1177180119828114

82. Hazel K, Mohatt G. Cultural and spiritual coping in sobriety: Informing substance abuse prevention for Alaska Native communities. *Journal of Community Psychology.* 2001;29(5):541–562.

83. McGregor D, Morelli P, Matsuoka J, Minerbi L. An ecological model of well-being. In: Becker HA, Vanclay F, eds. *The international handbook of social impact assessment: Conceptual and methodological advances.* Cheltenham, UK: Edward Elgar; 2003:109–126.

84. Mark GT, Lyons AC. Maori healers' views on wellbeing: the importance of mind, body, spirit, family and land. *Social Science & Medicine.* 2010;70(11):1756–1764.

85. Kahn-John M, Koithan M. Living in health, harmony, and beauty: the Dine (Navajo) Hózhó wellness philosophy. *Global Advances in Health and Medicine.* 2015;4(3):24–30.

86. Garroutte EM, Goldberg J, Beals J, Herrell R, Manson SM, AI-SUPERPFP Team. Spirituality and attempted suicide among American Indians. *Social Science & Medicine.* 2003;56(7):1571–1579.

87. Torres Stone RA, Whitbeck LB, Chen X, Johnson K, Olson DM. Traditional practices, traditional spirituality, and alcohol cessation among American Indians. *Journal of Studies on Alcohol and Drugs.* 2006;67(2):236–244.

88. Kulis S, Hodge DR, Ayers SL, Brown EF, Marsiglia FF. Spirituality and religion: Intertwined protective factors for substance use among urban American Indian youth. *The American Journal of Drug and Alcohol Abuse.* 2012;38(5):444–449.

89. Bear UR, Croy C, Kaufman C, Thayer Z, Manson S, AI-SUPERPFP Team. The relationship of five boarding school experiences and physical health status among Northern Plains Tribes. *Quality of Life Research.* 2018;27(1):153–157.

90. Gall A, Anderson K, Howard K, et al. Wellbeing of Indigenous Peoples in Canada, Aotearoa (New Zealand) and the United States: A systematic review. *International Journal of Environmental Research and Public Health.* 2021;18(11):1–31.

91. Wilson K. Therapeutic landscapes and First Nations peoples: An exploration of culture, health and place. *Health & Place.* 2003;9:83–93.

92. Shultz K, Cattaneo L, Sabina C, Brunner L, Jackson S, Serrata J. Key roles of community connectedness in healing from trauma. *Psychology of Violence.* 2016;6(1):42–48.

93. Simpson L. Indigenous environmental education for cultural survival. *Canadian Journal of Environmental Education.* 2002;7(1):13–25.

94. Biddle N, Swee H. The relationship between wellbeing and Indigenous land, language and culture in Australia. *Australian Geographer.* 2012;43(3):215–232.

95. Blackstock C. The emergence of the breath of life theory. *Journal of Social Work Values and Ethics.* 2011;8(1):1–16.

96. Vizenor G. *Survivance: Narratives of Native presence.* Lincoln, NE: University of Nevada Press; 2008.

97. IllumiNative. Accessed August 3, 2022. http://illuminative.org.

98. Fish J. OrigiNatives: Original digital stories from Native America. Accessed August 3, 2022. http://jillianfish.com/originatives.

99. Indigenous stories of strength. Accessed August 3, 2022. http://cih.jhu.edu/programs/indigenous-stories-of-strength.

100. Kirmayer LJ, Dandeneau S, Marshall E, Phillips MK, Williamson KJ. Rethinking resilience from Indigenous perspectives. *Canadian Journal of Psychiatry.* 2011;56(2):84–91. doi:10.1177/070674371105600203

101. Fish J, Syed M. Native Americans in higher education: An ecological systems perspective. *Journal of College Student Development.* 2018;59(4):387–403.

102. Smith LT. *Decolonizing methodologies: Research and Indigenous peoples.* Basingstoke, UK: Palgrave Macmillan; 2012.

103. Israel BA, Schulz AJ, Parker EA, Becker AB. Review of community-based research: Assessing partnership approaches to improve public health. *Annual Review of Public Health.* 1998;19(1):173–202. doi:10.1146/annurev.publhealth.19.1.173

104. Israel BA, Parker EA, Rowe Z, et al. Community-based participatory research: Lessons learned from the Centers for Children's Environmental Health and Disease Prevention Research. *Environmental Health Perspectives.* 2005;113(10):1463–1471. doi:10.1289/ehp.7675

105. Wallerstein N, Duran B. Community-based participatory research contributions to intervention research: The intersection of science and practice to improve health equity. *American Journal of Public Health.* 2010;100(S1):S40–S46. doi:10.2105/AJPH.2009.184036

106. Harding T, Oetzel J. Implementation effectiveness of health interventions for indigenous communities: A systematic review. *Implementation Science.* 2019;14(1):76. doi:10.1186/s13012-019-0920-4

107. Harding A, Harper B, Stone D, et al. Conducting research with tribal communities: Sovereignty, ethics, and data-sharing issues. *Environmental Health Perspectives.* 2012;120(1):6–10. doi:10.1289/ehp.1103904

108. Fisher PA, Ball TJ. Tribal participatory research: Mechanisms of a collaborative model. *American Journal of Community Psychology.* 2003;32(3–4):207–216. doi:10.1023/B:AJCP.0000004742.39858.c5

109. Around Him D, Andalcio Aguilar T, Frederick A, Larsen H, Seiber M, Angal J. Tribal IRBs: A framework for understanding research oversight in American Indian and Alaska Native communities. *American Indian and Alaska Native Mental Health Research.* 2019;26(2):72–95.

110. Hiraldo DV. "If you are not at the table, you are on the menu": Lumbee Government strategies under state recognition. *Native American and Indigenous Studies.* 2020;7(1):36. doi:10.5749/natiindistudj.7.1.0036

111. Hiraldo D, James K, Carroll SR. Case report: Indigenous sovereignty in a pandemic: Tribal codes in the United States as preparedness. *Frontiers in Sociology.* 2021;6:617995. doi:10.3389/fsoc.2021.617995

112. Garrison NA, Hudson M, Ballantyne LL, et al. Genomic research through an Indigenous lens: Understanding the expectations. *Annual Review of Genomics and Human Genetics.* 2019;20(1):495–517. doi:10.1146/annurev-genom-083118-015434

113. Carroll SR, Garba I, Plevel R, et al. Using Indigenous standards to implement the CARE principles: Setting expectations through tribal research codes. *Frontiers in Genetics.* 2022;13:1–10. doi:10.3389/fgene.2022.823309

114. Carroll SR, Plevel R, Jennings LL, et al. Extending the CARE Principles from tribal research policies to benefit sharing in genomic research. *Frontiers in Genetics.* 2022;13:1052620. doi:10.3389/fgene.2022.1052620

115. Hudson M, Garrison NA, Sterling R, et al. Rights, interests and expectations: Indigenous perspectives on unrestricted access to genomic data. *National Review of Genetics.* 2020;21(6):377–384. doi:10.1038/s41576-020-0228-x

116. Kukutai T, Taylor J. *Indigenous data sovereignty: Toward an agenda.* Canberra: Australian National University Press; 2016.

117. Walter M, Kukutai T, Carroll SR, Rodriguez-Lonebear D. *Indigenous data sovereignty and policy.* London: Routledge; 2021.

118. Nelson DJ, Madsen LD. Representation of Native Americans in US science and engineering faculty. *MRS Bulletin.* 2018;43(5):379–383. doi:10.1557/mrs.2018.108

8

Black Bodies, Black Health

Disrupting Structural Racism through Humanistic and Social Science Research

Enobong Hannah "Anna" Branch, Candace King, and Michelle Stephens

In December of 2021, a medical illustration of a Black fetus went viral, spawning multiple news articles and public discussions across social media among doctors and the general public.[1] The reaction was due to the rarity of medical representations of Black bodies as generalized figures for humanity, and the discussion highlighted the normalization of Whiteness within medical fields, even at the indiscriminate level of the images used in anatomy textbooks. One doctor created a Twitter poll asking others, "Have you ever seen a dark-skinned Black baby inside a pregnant mother illustrated in a medical text?"[2] Ninety-six percent of the 4,000-plus respondents said no, and this was not an aberration limited to this Twitter sample. Less than 4 percent of medical texts feature illustrations of non-White bodies, as one study performed by researchers at the University of Pennsylvania has shown (Adelekun et al. 2021). This base-level of representation, or more accurately the lack thereof, has implications for who and what we see as normative, what is characterized as well and unwell, and which bodies we value and which we do not. One Twitter commentator summarized the consequences of this aptly by saying, "Most of modern medicine doesn't consider anything but White men's anatomy and physiology, even today. Its structural racism

---

[1] Aliyah [@Liyahsworld_xo]. (2021, December 2). *I've literally never seen a black foetus illustrated, ever.* [Tweet]. Twitter. https://twitter.com/Liyahsworld_Fxo/status/1466463156386021385?s=20.

[2] Dr. Raven the Science Maven [@ravenscimaven]. (2021, December 3). *Have you ever seen a dark-skinned Black baby inside a pregnant mother illustrated in medical texts? Poll in the thread.* [Tweet]. Twitter. https://twitter.com/ravenscimaven/status/1466836756406300672?s=D20.

Enobong Hannah "Anna" Branch, Candace King, and Michelle Stephens, *Black Bodies, Black Health*. In: *Research to Action*. Edited by: Claire Gibbons and Alonzo L. Plough, Oxford University Press. © Robert Wood Johnson Foundation (2026). DOI: 10.1093/9780197819876.003.0009

that's so baked into the systems that often not even people embedded in them realize the harm they're propagating."[3]

Black Bodies, Black Health (BBBH), a one-year research project supported by the Robert Wood Johnson Foundation (RWJF), centered humanistic and social scientific fields to identify strategies needed to disrupt structural racism as a determinant of health and well-being. The project focused on articulating the racialization processes by which White bodies have become naturalized and Black bodies have been made invisible as figures of human health and well-being, and the consequences of such processes of representation. The ultimate goal was to identify various approaches that foundations and related funding organizations can take to target, catalyze, and support research that focuses, both in theory and method, on disrupting a broader cultural imagination of disease that signifies Black/minority bodies as sites of disorder. The representation of Black bodies as unwell is the result of both deeply entrenched historical processes and modern discourses, and has consequences for how systems and structures engage and respond to disease in ways that serve to undermine the well-being of Black and non-White patients.

The Historical Roots of Contemporary Health Inequity

The fact that it was Chidiebere Ibe's illustration of a Black fetus that sparked a viral conversation about the medical field's devaluation of Black bodies in the United States is apt, given the historical treatment of Black motherhood. As the 20th century dawned, so did a fledgling eugenics movement that aimed to mitigate societal ills (crime, poverty, and immoral acts such as promiscuity) through selective breeding. While eugenics has been discredited, and most recognize the harm of designating groups as "fit" and "unfit," this underlying logic has continued, both insidiously and at times directly, to inform the treatment of Black mothers (Dikötter 1998). The early 20th century saw the emergence of the birth control movement. There was initially great opposition to birth control among early 20th-century conservatives, but that was neutralized in part by a wider discourse that framed birth

---

[3] Cosmic Whore-er [@liquidfox1]. (2021, December 3). *Have you ever seen a dark-skinned Black baby inside a pregnant mother illustrated in medical texts? Poll in the thread.* [Tweet]. Twitter. https://twitter.com/liquidfox1/status/1466911126390665217?s=20.

control as a means of controlling Black women's fertility, whether its use was voluntary or compulsory (McDaniel 1996; Davis 1981; Roberts 1997).

As the 20th century continued, so did these efforts to control Black women's fertility. The massive assault on Black women's bodies has been described as the "New Jane Crow" to highlight the lack of discourse about, and the historical trajectory of, the oppression of Black women in particular (Jones and Seabrook 2017). There were many reasons for sterilizations, including population control as connected to stereotypes of Black motherhood, US welfare discourse, and practice for medical students at local universities (Ko 2016, Thomas 1998). US doctors routinely refused to deliver the babies of Black women and Medicaid recipients who had already borne two or more children unless they consented to sterilization, whereas under a concurrent practice, White and middle-class mothers who had not had "enough" children by a given age were *refused* sterilization (Davis 1981).[4]

Black women only received legal protection from coercive sterilization after the fallout resulting from the notorious 1973 sterilization of Minnie Lee Relf, a 14-year-old Black girl in Mississippi who was first administered Depo Provera, and was subsequently surgically sterilized, after social workers noticed that boys were hanging around her house and feared Minnie might become pregnant while her family received benefits (Nelson 2003). Because these procedures—which Relf and her impoverished and illiterate parents were not fully informed of—had been paid for with federal funds, President Nixon hurriedly banned the use of such funds for the sterilization of minors and the informed consent guidelines that we consider standard today were established.

While this change sought to protect Americans from unethical treatment by requiring their consent, the practice and utility of Blacks as subjects in medical experimentation has long been exploited. Beginning in 1932, the US Public Health Service recruited 662 poor rural Black sharecroppers in Macon County, Alabama, for the benefit of exploring the untreated course of syphilis, which at the time was referred to as "bad blood" (Brandt 1978, Brown 2017). Black sharecroppers were lied to and recruited because they were seen as expendable. They were informed that they would receive treatment for "bad blood" and free healthcare if they consented to the study. As of 1955, it was recorded that 30 percent of the participants died from the

---

[4] Doctors followed a rubric known as the "rule of 120," in which the product of a mother's age and number of births had to equal or exceed 120 before they could be considered for sterilization. For more, see Deardorff 2014.

study (Brandt 1978). When penicillin was made available as an option for treating syphilis, it was denied to participants in the study (Brandt 1978). This study shockingly went on until 1972 and spanned the Jim Crow period into the Civil Rights Movement.

About 18 years after the start of the Tuskegee syphilis study, Johns Hopkins University used the cells of Henrietta Lacks, a Black rural tobacco farmer from Virginia to create the polio vaccine, making advancements in disease research that led to the expansion of the biomedical industry (Skloot 2010). Henrietta Lacks' human cell line, referred to as HELA, was the world's first immortal cell line to live indefinitely outside of the body, and it is now bought and sold to laboratories across the nation. Cells from the cancerous tumor within her cervix were cut out months before she died from cervical cancer in 1951 without her knowledge or consent (Skloot 2010). While Lacks' cells were looked at as remarkable and prolific, as a Black woman she was treated as disposable and garnering her consent was unnecessary.

These well-known and egregious historical examples of the indiscriminate use of Black bodies and their body parts to find cures for diseases and vaccinations have imprints on contemporary health disparities that have not been fully appreciated. Blacks were viewed as expendable, explicitly devalued, and deemed not worthy of being consulted for consent, informed of risk, and more. Denying Blacks' full humanity enabled their harsh and brutal treatment, and racism justified this intentional harm of Black life. Even today, many doctors and nurses believe that Black patients have higher pain tolerance than Whites. We speak often of the deep suspicion that still characterizes the engagement of Blacks with the medical establishment today, but we do not often reflect on the practices within the American healthcare system that continue to normalize Whiteness and thereby characterize Black bodies as unwell.

The Path Forward

The deleterious effects of experiencing racism on the individual level are increasingly understood and damning—from shortened life expectancy to premature birth, racial discrimination kills (Chae et al. 2020, Braveman et al. 2021). Yet the impacts of structural racism, while acknowledged, are less understood (Gee and Ford 2011). There is a renewed call to focus on racism and abandon race, that is, to track and disrupt racial disparities but not reify differences amongst racial groups (Braveman and Dominguez 2021). While this work of envisioning disruption is not often the domain of health experts, it is the intellectual strength of the humanities and social sciences. The BBBH project brought together cross-disciplinary groups of experts to explore and unpack structural racism in service of creating equitable health outcomes, centering humanistic and social scientific approaches. We recognized and valued the different lens that each field brought to the study of health inequity and racism.

Humanistic scholars think about the development of age-old conceptions of race that ground population health disparities. They examine histories of this way of thinking as well as the systems that produce, reinforce, and reify this pattern of thought. Humanists make connections between the representation of health and well-being as racialized, represented in cultural forms, medical discourse, and narratives of individual behavior, and emphasize the ways in which all of these contribute to both the imagination and the development of disease. The cultural representation of disease, from news media to public commentary, influences how systems and structures respond. When the origin of disease is culturally represented and understood in the public mind as rooted in individual reckless behavior, resolution requires individuals taking personal responsibility. Whereas, when the origin of disease is understood to be in the mind—deviation rooted in susceptibility, it is understood culturally as a public health challenge, which requires state investment and public sympathy. Using this lens, we can see, for example, how locating the challenges of the crack epidemic as a problem of individual behavior rooted in recklessness, led to a different public response than the opioid crisis. The race of the users—predominately Black in the case of crack and often White, in the case of opioids—humanists and many others argue had everything to do with the way systems were mobilized or not to respond.

Social scientists often focus on how health disparities and differential treatment are embedded in structures and systems in the present, highlighting how an emphasis on personal responsibility misses the systems and structures that influence and shape human behavior or differentially condition the response of the medical establishment to treat it. In contrast, a biomedical approach emphasizes physiological factors often exclusively, then aggregates to describe patterns and disparities across groups, which has led to a focus on interventions in individual behavior and typing of racial/ethnic groups as well or unwell, for example, Black women and obesity. Physiological factors and health outcomes, however, cannot be understood absent the structural conditions that give rise to disparities across groups. We need to understand the connection between behavior and physiological outcomes, but we cannot treat behavior as the sole site of intervention. BBBH drew on the intellectual strength of the humanities and social sciences to focus on racism and envision disruption, identifying avenues for exploration and change to grapple with the structural roots of racial disparities. This strong interdisciplinary focus informed our recommendations regarding how funding programs can best intervene in supporting scholarship that aims to disrupt structural racism and increase health equity.

Insights and Research Directions

The interdisciplinary approach of Black Bodies, Black Health was exemplified in the research specialties of the project's primary investigators, a sociologist (Branch) and a literary and cultural critic and psychoanalyst (Stephens). The BBBH Steering Committee covered a range of areas of expertise, including public health, family medicine, sociology and psychology, and queer and cultural studies. This group identified key lines of inquiry and illustrated the kinds of frameworks that would inform the seed grantees and shape the research insights that emerged from BBBH. For example, psychologist Luis Rivera (Rutgers-Newark) argues that precisely because the impact of structural racism is often insidious, one missing research approach is the investigation of the role of implicit bias in health inequities. He asks, how does implicit bias at the level of where people live impact Black Americans who reside in these areas? What are the best approaches for reducing the harm of implicit bias at the level of context and environment?

Perry Halkitis, Dean of the School of Public Health at Rutgers, has led the charge in arguing for a definition of racism as a public health crisis, impacting the advancement of medicine and the policies, systems, and organizational structures that, by their very nature, perpetuate discrimination. Shawna Hudson, Professor and Research Division Chief in the Department of Family Medicine and Community Health at the Rutgers Robert Wood Johnson Medical School, recommends research that engages more fully with the science of implementation, which "engages process, actors, and actions in context and seeks to promote the adoption and integration of evidence-based practices, interventions and policies into routine healthcare and public health settings." As she continues: "Implementation science differs from intervention research in that it focuses testing and understanding the strategies used to implement evidence-based practices, rather than on intervention effectiveness. As we work to disrupt structural racism, we need to encourage action-based and participatory scientific practices that incorporate iterative, plan-do-study-act cycles to help us to understand and operationalize impactful interventions and processes in action."

Dawne Mouzon, a sociologist (Rutgers-New Brunswick) whose research seeks to identify and explain risk and protective factors for the physical and mental health of populations of African descent, notes a pattern in Robert Wood Johnson Foundation awards between 2005 and 2007 that focus on cultural competency interventions, such as teaching healthcare providers "cultural shortcuts" of race/ethnic minority groups and often implicitly identifying "culture" as the main cause of health behavior and outcomes. She draws attention instead to research on a new concept, structural competency, which emerged in 2014 from the work of Jonathan Metzl, MD, PhD (a physician, psychiatrist, and sociologist) and Helena Hansen, MD (a psychiatrist). Structural competency focuses on clinical skills but identifies institutional factors and policies that shape health inequities, while offering a theoretically informed framework to design healthcare interventions that seek to improve both health and healthcare outcomes for marginalized patients. For Mouzon, the shift from cultural competency to structural competency is analogous to the recognition that structural racism, rather than interpersonal racism, is a stronger root cause of health and social inequities, and therefore a funding focus on structural competency interventions would chart an important new research direction.

Carlos Decena, a cultural and queer studies scholar in Latino and Caribbean Studies, draws from his experience with the cultural politics of HIV/AIDS to emphasize the need to stay alert to the nuances of the politics of representation when addressing all issues concerned with illness and the way it is discussed. At the nexus between humanities-based research and the questions of Blackness and health lie, he argues, both biological and population-based factors implicated in addressing health challenges as well as the materiality of the meaning-making practices of representation developed around those very problems. In other words, while remaining centered in the experience of health and illness in Black communities, he urges us also to attend substantively to how these experiences are represented, since representation often shapes the questions asked, the evidence gathered, and the solutions proposed.

From the fall of 2021 through fall 2022, an interdisciplinary team of Rutgers researchers and thought leaders, informed by a broader array of disciplinary approaches in the humanities, identified frameworks in the human and social sciences that would be productive directions for research. Through seed projects, workshops to develop a shared understanding of "race" and "disruption," and a conference with national experts on race and health equity research, BBBH identified an exciting set of research directions to think with in regard to future funding of research, directions that can have a disruptive impact on our understanding of the impacts of structural racism on health outcomes.

Mapping Health Inequity: Project Scope and Structure

BBBH began by offering seed grants to incentivize humanists, social scientists, and biomedical researchers across Rutgers to engage in interdisciplinary work to explore and unpack structural racism in service of creating equitable health outcomes. External experts not only attended the August BBBH conference but also provided one-on-one feedback on position papers developed by the seed grantees. Drawing on existing research and taking a local frame grounded in New Jersey[5], grantees were asked to envision the work of disruption of structural racism, reimagining systems drawing from a range of fields and theoretical approaches. We were especially interested in two types of projects—humanities projects that drew the connections, historically and conceptually, between how understandings of race have directly and negatively impacted health treatments and outcomes in the United States; and social scientific or biomedical research projects that foregrounded the humanistic assumptions or implications of their work, were grounded in New Jersey, and focused on linking research in the following subject areas to broader questions of health and well-being: schools/education, poverty, child welfare, environmental justice, work/labor, housing, law enforcement, criminal justice, and penal reform, all of which we envision as the structural underpinnings of health inequities.

[5] Orfield, Gary, Jongyeon Ee, and Ryan Coughlan. *New Jersey's Segregraceated Schools: Trends and Paths Forward."* Los Angeles: University of California, 2017. https://files.eric.ed.gov/fulltext/ED577712.pdf

The seed grant program had four aims: (1) to identify Rutgers faculty members whose scholarship and expertise were tied to one of the dimensions of structural racism impacting health that we aimed to explore; (2) to spur the intentional translation of field-specific knowledge and cutting-edge research on vexing questions into digestible insights for the benefit of the general public; (3) to encourage the engagement of community members in producing knowledge on both the impact of structural racism and its solutions, incorporating humanistic and social scientific methods such as storytelling, ethnography, community curation and digital archiving; and (4) to develop a position paper that outlines the research promise, avenues for interdisciplinary exploration as well as possible policy solutions or interventions to reduce structural racism in their respective area. Fifteen Rutgers faculty (representing Rutgers Biomedical and Health Sciences, New Brunswick, Newark, and Camden) were awarded seed grants and paired with an external expert—a researcher who was not in their field—to promote cross-disciplinary exchange and deepen their insights. We identified four distinct clusters: Black Bodies, Physician Education, Environmental Racism, and The Carceral State that reflected the intellectual domains of the seed grantees' projects.

The Black Bodies research cluster embodies and encompasses the overarching themes of the BBBH project. These projects, led by BBBH co-lead Anna Branch and her research project manager, Candace King, delve into the dynamics of performance and health. In particular, they consider how Black health and well-being are impacted while at work. In both projects, work is considered in both the professional and physiological context. For example, Yana Rodgers, professor in the Department of Labor Studies and Employment Relations and faculty director of the Center for Women and Work, along with members of her research team, Debra Lancaster and Sarah Small, examine the occupational crowding of Black workers into frontline industries during the pandemic. As their study finds, Black women were at a higher risk for exposure to COVID-19 due to occupational segregation.[6] Unlike Black workers, White workers in New Jersey were able to withdraw from frontline industries at the onset of the pandemic, especially in healthcare support services. As a result, Rodgers and her team conclude, Black workers are occupationally crowded to the benefit of not only White

---

[6] APM Research Lab Staff. "The Color of the Coronavirus: COVID-19 Deaths by Race and Ethnicity in the U.S." APM Research Lab, September 2020. https://www.apmresearchlab.org/covid/deaths-by-race#black.

wages, but also White health. The Black Bodies research cluster also included Peter Economou, Assistant Professor of Applied Psychology and Director of Organizational Psychology Programs, and his research team members Alexander Gamble and Tori Glascock. Their research aims to better understand the health consequences of race-related stress (RRS) and its overall impact on Black bodies, including physiological and psychological. In particular, their study examines Black student-athletes' experiences of RRS while attending both predominantly White institutions (PWIs) and historically Black colleges and universities (HBCUs). In some instances, structural racism is painted as a problem that is only *seen*, not *felt*. Both projects speak to the physiological impact of structural health disparities on Black bodies. More concretely, both projects clearly outline the processes by which structural racism produces tangible harm in Black communities. Both the occupational and athletic arenas speak to the notion of Black performance and how Black workers and athletes are adversely affected as a result.

As previously discussed, the relationship between Black patients and the medical establishment has been quite contentious in the United States, evidenced by deep distrust in the initial response to COVID-19 vaccinations. Medical doctors shape conceptions about the body, as well as notions of harm and cure. The projects in the Physician Education research cluster, led by BBBH co-lead Michelle Stephens and Shawna Hudson, consider the relationship between patient and practitioner. For example, Pamela Brug, a medical doctor at Rutgers Robert Wood Johnson Medical School, and Juana Hutchinson Colas, an Associate Professor of Obstetrics and Gynecology, study how socioeconomic factors, such as race, ethnicity, age, sex, and gender, create compounding effects that impact the decisions patients make about their health and create a divide between patient and physician. Similarly, Johanna Schoen, professor of History, observes a related issue in her study of Black and Hispanic mothers whose children were admitted to the Neonatal Intensive Care Unit. As Schoen reports, there was a technical language barrier between the clinician and their parents, which not only affected how they understood the medical process but also alienated them from the physician. This technical oversight is also present in other areas of healthcare. Alexandria Bauer, Assistant Research Professor in the Center of Alcohol and Substance Abuse Studies and Applied Psychology, found this divide in the mental health sector as well. Bauer found that there were social judgments that often created a rift between mental health patients and physicians. Such stigmas, Bauer notes, have adverse effects that lead to misdiagnoses because the provider either underestimates or over-exaggerates their symptoms.

Societal institutions such as the medical field and higher education are key determinants in Black health. The projects in the Physician Education research cluster confront the structural challenges within medical institutions that perpetuate Black harm. Similarly, the projects in the Carceral State research cluster, led by Dawne Mouzon, Luis Rivera, and Perry Halkitis, undertake a critical examination of the criminal justice system as a total institution. The criminal justice system has a profound impact on the health and well-being of people who are incarcerated as well as their families, and the effects persist after release from institutionalization. These projects tackle the physiological effects of mass incarceration and police exposure. Take, for instance, Lauren Lyons, a doctoral student in the Department of Philosophy, whose study unearths the longstanding effects of the criminal legal system well beyond the prison cell. Lyons connects both pre-determinants and post-effects of health from incarceration. She points out that Black people with chronic diseases and serious mental illnesses are disproportionately likely to be incarcerated, and those without may even be subjected to those traumas both during and after incarceration. Lori Hoggard, an Assistant Professor of Psychology, delved into the physiological effects of incarceration in her investigation of how police exposure is biologically embedded in a sample of African American men residing in New Jersey. African Americans are also nearly four times more likely than White Americans to be killed by police officers, significantly more likely than White Americans to be killed while unarmed, and significantly more likely to be the targets of non-lethal police force (e.g., taser, pepper spray). Given these facts, Hoggard views racial inequities in policing as a linchpin of racial inequities in health. Ann Bagchi, an Associate Professor in the Rutgers Business School, along with her research team members Dwight Peavy and Anna Rivera, take this approach further as they target the implicit bias within law enforcement. In addressing the stigmas that police officers harbor toward Black men and women through structural-level reforms, Bagchi and her team believe there is an opportunity to enhance equity within New Jersey's criminal justice system. However, Maxine Davis, an Assistant Professor in the School of Social Work, offers another move to address the structural racist underpinnings of policing. In her study of Intimate Partner Violence/Domestic Violence (IPV/DV), Davis re-envisions the resources necessary to overcome the systemic factors that increase risk of harm. Her recommendation draws on the strengths of Black community members' creativity rather than the use of problem-centered approaches to address the social issue of IPV.

In the Physician Education and Carceral State clusters, seed grantees tackle the issue of implicit bias that perpetuates health disparities from a number of angles. The projects in the fourth and final research cluster, Environmental Racism, led by Carlos Decena, are no different. All spaces are not created equal; studies have shown that standards of living vary by zip code, and where we live impacts how we live. These projects explore how the environment, including considerations of climate as well as other factors of space, impact health and well-being. A study on Black women and breast cancer screening led by Mei Fu, Senior Associate Dean of Nursing Research and Professor at the Rutgers–Camden (School of Nursing), and Wanda Williams, an Associate Professor of Nursing at the University of North Carolina, Greensboro (formerly of Rutgers–Camden), unveils the structural challenges that lead to health inequity. Fu, the principal investigator of the project, and Williams uncovered place-based structural and racial determinants such as transport and childcare needs that impede Black women's access to adequate care. Fu and Williams offer a unique approach to measuring the environmental factors that perpetuate health disparities. In the same vein, Anita Bakshi, an Assistant Professor of Teaching in the Department of Landscape Architecture, advocates for researchers to consider how individual stories can help to explicate the structural roots of racial disparities and health outcomes. For example, in her study of the Ramapough Turtle Clan, Bakshi writes that the Ramapough already have knowledges about their community health and its relation to the pollution of their land. Rachel Devlin, an Associate Professor of History, also argues for more scholarly consideration of the personal history of the people native to a region. In her study of "Cancer Alley," the "chemical corridor" stretching along the Mississippi River from Baton Rouge to New Orleans, Devlin highlights the storytelling of Amos Favorite, a pollution activist. She envisions his stories as valuable historical, numerical, local, and statistical data that researchers can rely on to highlight Black experiences of living with toxic pollution.

Together, the four BBBH research clusters helped us to identify three primary challenges in the study of Black Health:

1) Studying race: What does it mean to adequately address and attend to race within health disparities? How does race as a body of measurement, of difference, show up structurally?

2) Documenting harm: Harm is not a "one-time" or "one-size" instance. How do we identify, catalog, and address harm in a way that not only addresses the shortcomings of the structure, but also provides specific reprieve to those affected?

3) Limitations of researchers: Instances of gatekeeping prohibit certain research from being conducted and published and there are certain barriers to doing the work (i.e., money and time). What do researchers, and especially researchers of color, up and down the academic pipeline, need to carry out their work?

Project Findings and Initial Recommendations

The introduction to the Culture of Health Series' edited anthology, *Necessary conversations: Understanding racism as a barrier to achieving health equity*, begins with the plight of Jackson, Mississippi, whose residents were devastated by March 2020's record-breaking floods. This climate tragedy left inhabitants, who are predominantly Black, without safe drinking water. Two years later, Jackson was still facing a dry well from the city officials' negligence, with the Justice Department issuing a warning that "an imminent and substantial endangerment to human health exists" (Harris et. al 2022). As the nearly three year-long battle for clean water conveys, the health inequities within Black communities like Jackson are not only pervasive, but persistent. The Black Bodies, Black Health External Expert Conference held on August 16–18, 2022 represented an effort to unpack the compounding effects that lead to inequity and to help envision a path forward to develop an ecosystem tailored to advance racial and health equity. As Robert Wood Johnson Foundation (RWJF) Chief Science Officer and Vice President of Research-Evaluation-Learning Alonzo Plough asserts in *Necessary conversations*, "a Culture of Health is impossible without a full-bore commitment to racial equity." With this commitment in mind, seed grantees met one-on-one with external experts and their research cluster as a whole to discuss challenges and offer recommendations for agencies and foundations invested in furthering research impact in race and health equity.[7]

---

[7] Plough, Alonzo L., ed. *Necessary Conversations: Understanding Racism as a Barrier to Achieving Health Equity.* New York: Oxford University Press, 2022. https://www.rwjf.org/en/insights/our-research/2022/05/necessary-conversations--we-need-to-talk-about-race-health-and-equity.html

General Recommendations from Cross Cluster Insights

An annual Black Bodies, Black Health convening and/or active BBBH working group: A majority of seed grantees and external experts expressed the value of a forum, such as BBBH and a strong interest in returning to develop their projects, while engaging with public actors on the issue of health inequity.

Meeting among community and other local actors in New Jersey: Many felt that inviting government officials, community organizers and educators, and health physicians to the conversation might help them to benefit more directly from research that envisions anew what the future could be.

Fund projects that would not only serve a scholarly purpose, but also support researchers: There is a need for funding opportunities that are process-oriented (e.g., creating space for researchers' thinking and thinking together), that can support research projects in the early stages of conceptualization and development.

Specific Research Cluster Recommendations and Insights

Black Bodies

For the researchers working and dialoguing together in this cluster, systemic challenges to their research included: the lack of shared language in the study of Black bodies, insufficient attention paid to how race shows up structurally, and the inadequacy of systems for Black workers that have been set up to support well-being. Research findings included evidence of systemic oppression within athletic systems and the long-term deleterious effects of those systems on Black student athletes, including physiological markers of stress. Findings also revealed the negative effects of occupational crowding of Black workers into frontline industries during the pandemic.

To ameliorate these research and socio-historical challenges, researchers called for increased funding for critical thinking spaces, that is, funding for more spaces and convenings to think about the historical and cultural processes that produce our narratives about the Black body, and to create further opportunities for collaboration across disciplines. Researchers also argued more specifically for better financial support and comprehensive health training for athletic departments, entailing infrastructures in which athletic departments engage in educational experiences and self-reflection on how their actions and words may aid in the oppression and commodification of Black student-athletes. They also recommended funding for more targeted efforts to collect community survey data on the experiences of Black workers in essential jobs, gauging their health risks and the extent to which workplace supports alleviate those risks, including in collective bargaining, in education and training programs, and in stronger care infrastructures.

The Black Bodies research cluster focused on health inequities that occur at the margins and intersections of social identity. Black Bodies cluster participants agreed that "health" is experienced in a myriad of ways as it relates to harm or cure; therefore, when addressing health, they argued that we must attend to the intersections of Black identity (i.e., class, sexuality, faith, etc.). To examine these theoretical ideas in practice, participants were interested in developing shared language across disciplines and breaking down silos across fields such as economics, biostatistics, public health, and sociology. For example, social and behavioral sciences (economics and sociology) widely use "time use surveys" to highlight the unequal burden that women bear for the second shift in the home, using real-time information on the activities of men and women to document gender inequality. Public health/biostatistics researchers widely use "ecological measurement assessment" to gather real-time information on health behavior. Economist Yana Rodgers and external expert Stephanie Cook had an enlightening conversation when they realized the potential of linking these two data forms in future data collection strategies to make the structural impact of health inequity more visible. The discovery of such methodological affinities across disciplines might offer useful frameworks for understanding health at the margins.

The participants reflected on a number of barriers and blind spots that researchers face while carrying out their work, one of which includes gatekeeping and funding. Creating funding incentives for scholars to carry out interdisciplinary work on health disparities is crucial, as field-stretching innovations are not often encouraged on the tenure track and beyond. Critical insights into our understanding of the impact of racism on health at the structural and system levels occur when we invest and spend time in dialogue to understand our disciplinary lanes and purposefully push the boundaries. More opportunities for disciplines to engage with one another in the interest of disrupting health disparities across multiple domains would be immensely beneficial for the field. As disciplines come together to address pressing issues, we can better engage public actors, organizations, and health practitioners to collectively advance change.

Physician Education

Researchers found that certain systemic challenges set the context for the inadequate education of physicians and healthcare professionals in understanding the relationships between racism and healthcare equity. Minority access to proper healthcare, sub-par care received by many members of ethnic minority populations, barriers for minorities to seeking healthcare as a profession, and "one-size fits all" and colorblind approaches to care, all negatively impacted patients of color and their relationships to the medical and healthcare industry.

Researchers called strongly for comprehensive training for healthcare providers to recognize the non-monolithic nature of the populations that they serve. They also called for increased support for Black clinicians on the pathway and retention pipeline into the medical field—beginning in elementary school, well before traditional high school and college prep programs. Such initiatives would show communities that the healthcare and public health work opportunities and center on making other clinical tracks, beyond the MD, visible as options for Black youth (e.g., nursing, physician assistants, social work, behavioral health, etc.). Researchers also felt that there was a strong need for community engagement and participatory action-based research. We should be addressing community, patient, and healthcare system research needs by advancing research designs that move beyond traditional approaches currently valued in many fields (i.e., hypothesis-driven and RCT studies).

Overall, the participants in the Physician Education research cluster recommended shifting the discussion of and research approaches to healthcare in the United States from the purely biomedical to the biopsychosocial. Such an approach will require that providers, particularly medical providers, attend to the psychological, psychosocial, social, and structural factors that shape help in the delivery of service. Attending to health in this manner will in turn empower patients to speak openly about their life experiences, including the experiences of systemic racism that adversely affect their health and well-being. In order to enact change in the health disparities noted across populations that are marginalized and oppressed, there must be ongoing and consistent training for providers during their disciplinary studies, including but not limited to open and clear conversations about implicit biases and stereotype threat.

It was also suggested that there must be an ongoing effort to create avenues for racial minorities to pursue healthcare as a profession. This requires not only addressing the economic disparities faced by members of racial minority groups but also shifting the sensibilities and assumptions of the health professions, particularly medicine, to the paradigm reviewed above that disparages the Black body. With regard to research, efforts must be undertaken to develop and test interventions that support health equity. It was clear that there is a substantive body of literature on health disparities across race. While documenting these disparities has been key, it is imperative that the dialogue shift to enacting health inequity. This entails studies that move beyond the overly simplistic delineation of disparities across demographic states, including but not limited to race.

The Carceral State

For the researchers in this cluster, systemic challenges included Black hypervisibility in the criminal justice system and in fatal encounters with police, the direct and indirect consequences of the criminal legal system on incarcerated people and their families (such as the interruption of education, the strain on family networks, and destabilizing housing), and a policymaking process that inflicts trauma and stress on the wider community.[8]

To address these challenges, researchers recommended more effective training for police officers to mitigate implicit bias within the criminal justice system, building better data to avoid overreliance on racial statistics and the reification of differences between racial groups, and investing in community empowerment models so that affected communities have a voice in the process, with creative community designed and led solutions that offer specific interventions as opposed to "one-size" approaches. Funding research studies that explore other systems of social support (i.e., the provisions of housing, food, healthcare, etc. to disrupt the root causes of crime and structural injustice/racism) was determined to be key, in addition to funding for research that evaluates policy to address the need for racial impact assessments for all new and existing legislation. Research must be prioritized that evaluates specific interventions (i.e., policies, programs, practices) that

---

[8] Massoglia, Michael. 2008. "Incarceration, Health, and Racial Disparities in Health." *Law & Society Review* 42.2 (2008): 275–306. doi:10.1111/j.1540-5893.2008.00342.x

have the potential to counteract the harms of structural racism and improve health, well-being, and equity outcomes.

This research cluster engaged in a lively discussion about how funding agencies should change their funding priorities. For example, for community-based participatory research, they should expand their notion of who is a "legitimate researcher" (such as funding community members/organizations to collect their own big data because they are experts in their own right). Research should be done "Not about us without us," a key phrase used to justify the need for true community partnership. Participants also shared the need for funding projects that allow space for thinking, amplifying the need above for developing funding opportunities that are process-oriented (e.g., collaborative development), as opposed to fully developed research projects. Participants shared the ethos that it was "necessary to yield creative disruption." Research is not just science, it is about other types of production as well. Most participants acknowledged that this is also a constraint in their own disciplines and institutions (i.e., the thinking process is not prioritized in terms of tenure and/or promotion). One external expert called for the funding of future "thought leaders" and encouraged more "thought leadership systems."

Environmental Racism

In the research area of environmental racism, especially as it pertains to communities and women of color, systemic challenges include: the healthcare barriers related to place-based structural and racial determinants; a lack of support by major national agencies that currently do not support, for example, breast self-examination (BSE); uncomfortable mammogram procedures that induce pain and tenderness; and the discomfort felt by some Black women patients, who found their technicians to be unpleasant and uncaring. All of these can discourage preventive screenings. The lack of forums for community stories to be told and heard compounds the physical harm and illnesses community members live with.

To address and disrupt these challenges, researchers recommended mitigating environmental barriers to healthcare access by meeting needs and alleviating hardships, such as transportation and childcare, and extending hours of mammogram screening on evenings and weekends for Black and minority women. Researchers described the need for ongoing education and encouragement of breast self-examinations among Black women. Expanding the definition of data would allow researchers to look for "measurements" in atypical patient accounts that fall outside of those provided by the medical establishment and agencies like the CDC, such as native storytelling. Research that prioritizes local voices, how local and community stories can help to explicate the structural roots of racial disparities and health outcomes, would be an important new direction in health disparities research.

The discussion of the Ramapough Lunaape Nation Turtle Clan's projects in particular, concerning their resignifications of food sovereignty and relationship to land in the context of environmental degradation, offered an opportunity for a wide-ranging discussion of cultural politics and expressive praxis in relation to shifting views and political work in health in indigenous and Black communities. A dimension of the "public-facing" nature of this work was demonstrated in how the researchers accompanied the Turtle Clan's efforts to generate alternative histories, representations, and claims related to their lands and how they link land contamination to the illnesses they experience. While it remains important to question and challenge the power-laden interactions shaping the research encounter, the conversation generated by this project put a stronger emphasis on the value that research can have in producing resources for communities actively engaged in cultural struggle. Thus, what is being reimagined here is not just research as "public-facing" work but the function of research in community. Rejecting an extractive ethos, work of this kind instead turns into the production artifacts that the community can mobilize in their efforts to raise awareness and combat environmental degradation. Interaction with the grantees, their mentors, and members of other clusters brought attention to the possibility that what we are incubating, collectively, is a different way to imagine the function of research.

Insights from the Research Process

BBBH began with a simple question on research process: What would we learn from bringing humanists, social scientists, and biomedical researchers to the table to explore, unpack, and disrupt structural racism in service of creating equitable health outcomes? What would a just racial future require to remediate the imprints of the past in the structures of our present? The structure of interaction around these research questions, framings, findings, and next steps was, itself, an original creation emerging from this process. In most grant/grantee settings, funds are disbursed with the expectation of a product and perhaps some "check points" with program officers. The fact that this process was structured with a "heavier hand," so to speak, with seed grantees required to be in substantive engagement with the leaders of the project, with external experts, and with each other, created something of much greater value.

In the three-day August conference, for example, the question of "tenderness" in the treatment of Black women in breast cancer screening encounters produced a conversation that extended far beyond the feedback the seed grantee received. Together, the participants of the cluster conversation touched on questions of the clinical encounter itself, how it is embedded (or not) in communities of care, how Black women experience the biomedical encounter as alienating both as racialized and classed subjects in Camden, New Jersey, and how we factor in the "local" in thinking about race and health. As the discussion spread over the two days of the meeting, the cluster came back to these points with additional insights and questions for the researchers, and many noted just how rare it is to have research in progress treated in this way.

Other key insights emerged from the process overall. One constant topic over the course of this research process was how to study race in a way that moves away from reifying race. Reimagining race at the individual level (interpersonal perceptions of race and experiences with racism), and at a structural level (involving both racist systems and histories) revealed the power of research questions and approaches in which these two factors are not held as mutually exclusive. To reimagine race, one cannot isolate the individual from the places and communities in which they live and work. Places are imbued with systems, including those that are racist and racializing, but they are also imbued with racist individuals from high status groups who create, maintain, and protect the systems. How do you deploy race and disrupt racism without simultaneously reifying race in both individuals and systems? One important outcome of the BBBH project has been this understanding of the necessary intersection between individuals and places, and its broader implications for health inequities. To reimagine race and its effect on Black bodies and Black health, scholarship and research should adopt intersectional approaches.

Another topic emerged as grantees grappled with the operationalization and measurement of race, particularly in some of their disciplines. What are we talking about when we refer to race, racism, and even systemic racism? How does one measure race and racism today when the demography of the United States is changing so rapidly? Most individuals are comfortable with identifying with prevailing racial categories, but do these racial categories "accurately" represent the individuals who fall into them? How do we disrupt these long-standing categories that often hinder our understanding of Black bodies and Black health? These questions are particularly significant in the carceral state, where justice-involved individuals are often seen through a racialized lens (i.e., the racialization of bodies), undermining the basic humanity of these same individuals. How do we measure race in the carceral state to achieve a just future?

Community was another theme that often came up in cluster discussions. What roles do community and the community play, if any, in the effect of the carceral state on Black bodies and Black health? Do communities that are affected by system racism understand that racism is a key barrier to leveraging their strengths to problem solve? Clearly communities need to be engaged, but how do we move a community from cohesion to mobilization to effect change in the carceral state? How does a community make the case of race and racism to policymakers, and influence equitable policy? Should communities hold the carceral state accountable or responsible? The carceral state is supposed to be a space of rehabilitation, but one sense emerging from this project is that this is less possible when community involvement and initiatives are not encouraged.

Over the course of two workshops and a conference with external experts, the BBBH leads, steering committee, and seed grantees came to a shared internal understanding of the goals, challenges and possibilities of our work together. Overall, an important takeaway of the BBBH experience was the value of this kind of intellectual stewardship as crucial to the "incubation" of research on racialized health disparities.

Appendix

The first BBBH workshop focused on developing a shared vocabulary of race across fields and the second identified themes and introduced field vexing questions that emerged from the respective seed projects. The workshops were followed by an external expert conference that aimed to tell a cross-cutting story of the BBBH project privileging four factors: the centering of the black body, tracing the history of cultural representations of the Black body in European and American culture, defining structural racism as itself a public health issue, and mapping the geographical determinants of race and health outcomes as a question of value. We used a graphical illustrator to visually capture key ideas in real time. The graphical illustrations recorded by our sketch effect artist, Joe Watkins, and generated from these convenings are included in this appendix.

The first illustration (Figure A.1) captures the seed grantees' descriptions and discussions of their conceptualizations of their projects. A continuous point of discussion in the second workshop, and throughout the BBBH project, was the conceptualization of disruption. What does disruption mean and how useful is the word disruption? The unresolved tension between reimagining and reifying race emerged as central to the goal of disruption.

The remaining graphical illustrations (Figures A.2–A.5) were generated from four prompting talks held as part of the external expert conference.

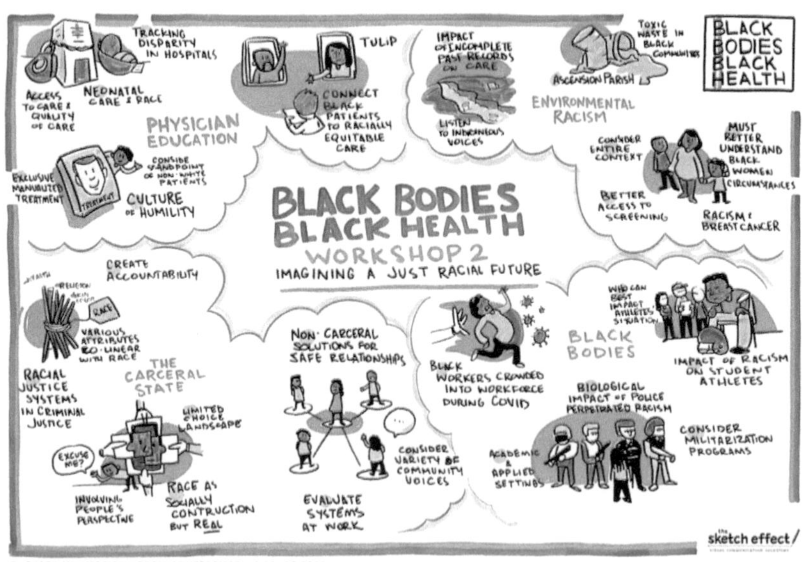

Figure A.1   Second BBBH Workshop on disruption

The graphical illustrator from the BBBH external expert workshop used a video recording to create this image.

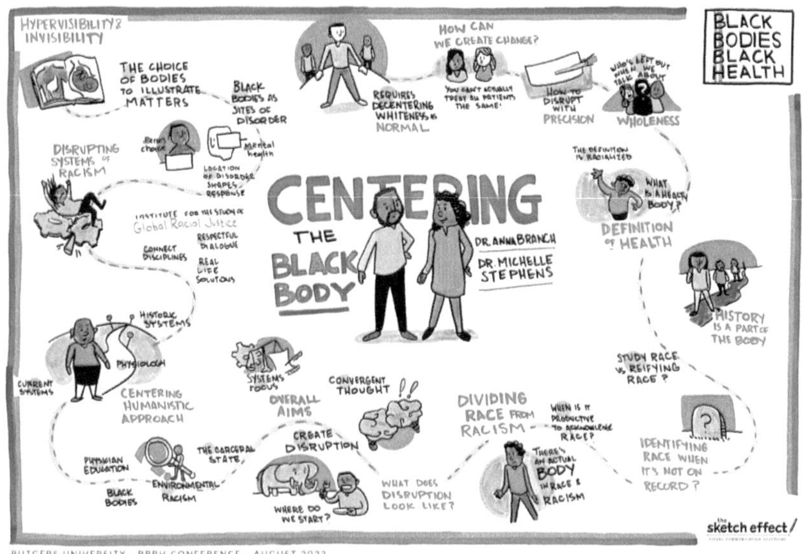

Figure A.2 Drs. Branch and Stephens opening prompting talk at external expert conference

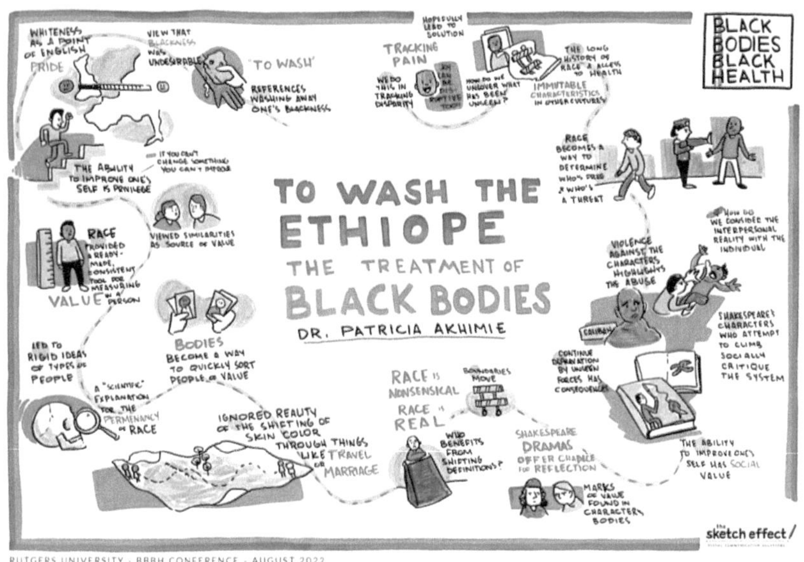

Figure A.3 Prompting talk by Dr. Patricia Akhimie

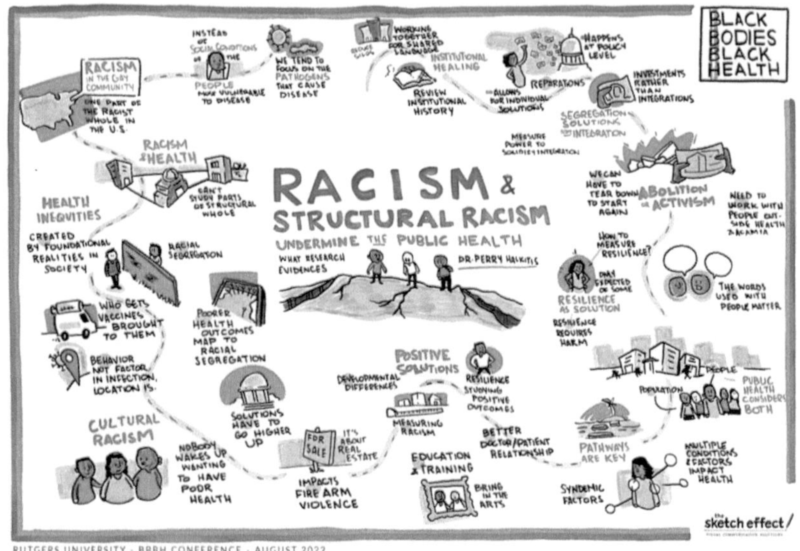

Figure A.4 Prompting talk by Dean Perry Halkitis

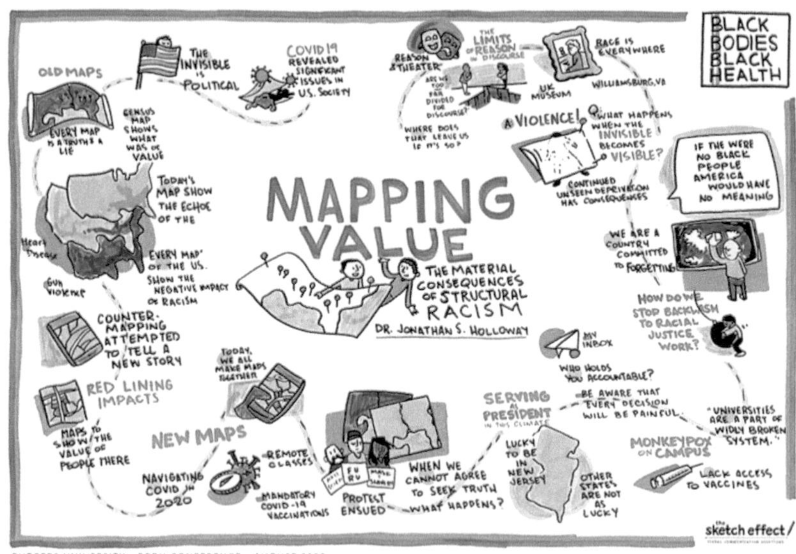

Figure A.5 Presidential keynote by Dr. Jonathan S. Holloway

They highlight takeaways from the opening address by project co-leads Drs. Anna Branch and Michelle Stephens, a presidential keynote by Rutgers President Dr. Jonathan S. Holloway, a presentation on the narrative origins of the disparate treatment of Black bodies by Associate Professor of English, Dr. Patricia Akhimie, and a presentation on how racism and structural racism undermine the public health by Dean of the School of Public Health, Dr. Perry Halkitis.

All prompting talks at the BBBH Conference, including the presidential keynote, were recorded and publicly available for viewing on demand on the ISGRJ website. To access the full conversation, please review the following link on our YouTube page: https://www.youtube.com/watch?v=2584 YapyiHg

References

Adelekun, Ademide, Ginikanwa Onyekaba, and Jules B. Lipoff. "Skin Color in Dermatology Textbooks: An Updated Evaluation and Analysis." *Journal of the American Academy of Dermatology* 84.1 (2021): 194–196.

Brandt, Allan M. "Racism and Research: The Case of the Tuskegee Syphilis Study." *Hastings Center Report* 8.6 (1978): 21–29.

Braveman, Paula, et al. "Explaining the Black-White Disparity in Preterm Birth: A Consensus Statement from a Multi-disciplinary Scientific Work Group Convened by the March of Dimes." *Frontiers in Reproductive Health* 3 (2021): 49.

Braveman, Paula, and Tyan Parker Dominguez. "Abandon 'race.' Focus on Racism." *Frontiers in Public Health* 9 (2021): 1318.

Brown, DeNeen L. "'You've got bad blood': The Horror of the Tuskegee Syphilis Experiment." *The Washington Post*, May 16, 2017.

Chae, David H et al. "Racial Discrimination and Telomere Shortening among African Americans: The Coronary Artery Risk Development in Young Adults (CARDIA) Study." *Health Psychology: Official Journal of the Division of Health Psychology* 39.3 (2020): 209–219. doi:10.1037/hea0000832

Davis, Angela Y. *Women, Race, & Class*. New York: Vintage Books, 1981.

Deardorff, Julie. "Doctors Reluctant to Give Young Women Permanent Birth Control." *The Chicago Tribune*, May 13, 2014.

Dikötter, Frank. "Race Culture: Recent Perspectives on the History of Eugenics." *The American Historical Review* 103.2 (1998): 467–478.

Gee, Gilbert C., and Chandra L. Ford. "Structural Racism and Health Inequities: Old Issues, New Directions." *Du Bois Review* 8.1 (2011):115–132. doi: 10.1017/S1742058X11000130

Harris, Bracey, Zinhle Essamuah, and Phil McCausland. "Justice Department Steps in Amid Warnings that Jackson's Water System Is at a 'Breaking Point,'" *NBC News*, September 27, 2022.

Jones, Chenelle A., and Renita L. Seabrook. "The New Jane Crow: Mass Incarceration and the Denied Maternity of Black Women." In: Deflem, Mathieu, ed. *Race, Ethnicity and Law*. Bingley, UK: Emerald Publishing Limited, 2017: 135–154.

Ko, Lisa. "Unwanted Sterilization and Eugenics Programs in the United States." *PBS Independent Lens*, January 29, 2016.

McDaniel, Antonio. "Fertility and Racial Stratification." *Population and Development Review* 22 (1996): 134–150.

Nelson, Jennifer. *Women of Color and the Reproductive Rights Movement*. New York: NYU Press, 2003.

Roberts, Dorothy. *Killing the Black Body: Race, Reproduction, and the Meaning of Liberty*. New York: Vintage Books, 1997.

Skloot, Rebecca. *The Immortal Life of Henrietta Lacks*. New York: Broadway Paperbacks, 2010.

Thomas, Susan L. "Race, Gender, and Welfare Reform: The Antinatalist Response." *Journal of Black Studies* 28.4 (1998): 419–446.

9

Centering Health Equity and Community Voice in Climate Change

By Jennifer Messenger, Tori O'Neal, and Surili Sutaria Patel With: Erica Ellis, Eric Friedenwald-Fishman, Max Friedenwald-Fishman, Shadiin Garcia, Kirsten Gunst, Kelly Hilovsky, Aayaan Jamwal, Kevin Kirkpatrick, Thomas Price Lang, and Vernice Miller-Travis

"[W]ithout racial justice, communities of color will never achieve the health outcomes that [our communities are] hoping for."

—Interviewee

The Robert Wood Johnson Foundation (RWJF) is focusing its resources and energy directly toward dismantling structural racism to improve health outcomes. The quote above, from one of the interviews with community-based leaders that anchor this chapter, captures the spirit, hope, and expectation that many people we interviewed expressed. The health outcomes this interviewee and many others envision for communities of color include thriving, not mere survival or resilience; the ability to envision and create a desired future; and the opportunity to reap the benefits of living in the United States and in tribal nations rather than merely bearing the burdens. This means people must be free from stress, trauma, disease, and death at the hands of structural racism.

This chapter is an exploration rooted in community experience, expertise, and wisdom. It complements the other chapters contributed here and adds the vital voices of people whose lived experience and professional work are anchored in communities most impacted by structural racism, colonization, and oppression, and who absolutely must be at the forefront of identifying urgent needs and defining priority actions.

Jennifer Messenger, Tori O'Neal, and Surili Sutaria Patel, *Centering Health Equity and Community Voice in Climate Change*. In: *Research to Action*. Edited by: Claire Gibbons and Alonzo L. Plough, Oxford University Press. © Robert Wood Johnson Foundation (2026). DOI: 10.1093/9780197819876.003.0010

As a social impact organization with expertise in public health, environmental sustainability, and social justice, Metropolitan Group brings a shared commitment to health equity and racial justice. Further, we understand how structural racism contributes to climate change, in particular, by rewarding extractive use of and inequitable access to resources. And we understand how structural racism exacerbates the health impact of climate change in communities of color and Indigenous communities in myriad ways: it influences where people live, raises intentional barriers to resources to endure climate disasters, and increases exposure to risk due to overrepresentation in frontline jobs.

In this chapter, we offer objective findings followed by our analysis and recommendations. We are honored to be trusted with the stories and insights that inform the findings we offer here.

Methodology

Our team of researchers, social change agents, and subject matter specialists in racial justice, health, climate, narrative, and other fields designed our research methodology to answer three questions:

1. What is the evidence for actions to address structural racism and improve health outcomes?
2. What specific considerations exist for potential action at the intersection of climate change, structural racism, and health?
3. What are the narratives shaping these issues, and what role might the Foundation play in narrative change?

To find the answers, we combined three modes of inquiry, as set out below.

Community-Informed Literature Review

To complement RWJF's large-scale academic research review, we conducted a parallel review of community-informed literature: both academic and gray literature (e.g., blog posts, papers, press releases, videos, research, and other evidence offered outside traditional academic circles and paywalls) designed, researched, delivered, and owned by people from and working in communities of color and Indigenous communities.

Typical literature review methodologies too often exclude these voices, prioritizing access to and credentials from academia. We are not discounting the important contributions of Black and Brown researchers in journals and high-level research institutions; rather, we are committing to a broader set of sources, with a more inclusive definition of expert and evidence that values lived experience, community action, and local wisdom.

We focused the literature review on evidence for actions to address the intersection of climate change, structural racism, and health. To reflect current conditions and contemporary solutions, a majority of the sources we considered were published since 2019. We identified sources through Duck-DuckGo using a variety of search terms. We narrowed the initial yield of 84 sources to 35 final sources and five case studies.

The literature review provided insights into recent actions and strategies that are being used most often to create change, offering evidence of what is working and may benefit from additional investment and capacity. Communities, local businesses, governments, and others, working in collaboration, are identifying solutions. They crave the skills and capacity to implement creative interventions to improve the health of families.

Interviews with Community-Grounded and Recognized Leaders

We identified and prioritized a wide range of activists, advocates, influencers, researchers, funders, and others from and working in communities experiencing structural racism using the following criteria:

- Has expertise and perspective on structural racism's impact on health, and, for at least one-third of interviewees, climate justice expertise.
- Is nationally or regionally recognized in their area of focus by the communities they serve or represent.
- Has run or is running an organization or campaign within their area of focus.
- Is recognized by the grasstops within their area of focus.

- Is actively engaged in addressing structural racism.
- A range of geography, race and ethnicity, gender identity, and age.

Nineteen of 30 potential interviewees accepted. Interviews included one-to-one sessions and small groups.

The interviewees represent decades of direct experience working to dismantle structural racism. They bring expertise and wisdom on changes and solutions that are effective or have impact and those that are not. Stories, direct experience, and community-informed inputs are data that carry weight equal to—and complement—academic literature and other forms of evidence.

Scan of Narratives and Evidence-Informed Narrative Actions

Building on the Foundation's interest and investments in narrative change as a lever of change, we explored narratives advancing and hindering efforts to address structural racism and improve health. Our exploration included three components:

1. A scan of 31 documents, including messaging and narrative guides on structural racism and health—integrating climate change where possible—as well as articles and reports on effective narrative action to address these issues.
2. Narrative questions in the interviews, plus a handful of interviews with people focused on narrative change.
3. A cursory social media scan to surface dominant productive and counterproductive themes.

Limitations

The greatest limitations were those of timing and scale. We attempted to be as broad in our review as possible, within our three-month window and approved scope.

As a social justice-focused firm, we acknowledge that we enter this research with a distinct point of view. To guard against confirmation bias, we engaged a broad team in the work and a separate team of reviewers and analysts.

Findings

In this section, we offer objective topline findings representing key themes across the research.

Finding 1: When Structural Racism Is the Core Problem, Priority Actions Are the Same no Matter the Issue

We asked all interviewees, including climate and environmental justice experts, "What is the evidence for actions to address structural racism and improve health outcomes? What is the evidence for actions at the intersection of climate change, structural racism, and health?"

In almost all cases, answers to both questions were the same: Until we as a society address structural racism—the structures that hold oppression in place and allow the notion of disposable people to persist—we cannot make progress on any issue.

Additionally, as we scanned the literature for priority actions, we found that they were less specific about climate and more about *how* the work is done in community, emphasizing community power, movement building, and self-determination—the themes that surfaced in the interviews.

The solutions to curb climate change and its impact on health overlap with solutions to dismantle structural, institutional, and environmental racism. Thus, we have one core set of findings for evidence of vital actions to take to address structural racism, aligned with any specific issue, to improve health outcomes.

Finding 2: Addressing Structural Racism to Improve Health Demands a Sharp Focus on Structures

Structures define access and processes, determine who has power and who does not, and restrict seats at the decision-making table. The need to work at a structural level came up often, with emphasis on four primary structures: 1) electoral justice, 2) economic justice, 3) power and decision-making authority, and 4) narrative.

1. Electoral Justice

Electoral justice is foundational, interviewees said; without it, no other structures can shift.

According to a recent report by the de Beaumont Foundation, there is clear evidence connecting civic engagement with improved health and racial equity: "When larger numbers of people from certain communities and groups participate in voting, it translates into greater influence over determining who holds political power to advance policies that respond to the needs and priorities of their community. Thus, voting drives the policies that shape the social determinants of health and equity" (de Beaumont Foundation 2021).

> "There is no pathway to eliminating structural inequalities and positively impacting health and wellbeing in marginalized communities—and definitely in the Black community—without policy changes. And the path to policy changes is paved by civic engagement. Communities cannot engage civically without full and unfettered access to the ballot box."
>
> —Interviewee

For Black and Indigenous communities, as well as all other communities of color, however, exercising the right to vote in the United States is becoming increasingly more difficult—and in some cases physically unsafe. With the Voting Rights Act severely weakened by the Supreme Court *Citizens United* decision, key voter protections are no longer in place for all.

Citizens exercising their right to vote elect leaders at the local, state, and national levels who then go on to enact the policies and regulations that govern the United States. *They control the structures.* For this reason, nearly every interviewee lifted up electoral justice as an area of great need in which the Foundation should significantly engage.

2. Economic Justice

> "[T]he lost wealth of Black Americans—the stolen wealth over several generations—directly contributed to significant health disparities for Black people in the U.S., and … this needs to be acknowledged and addressed."
>
> —Interviewee

Economic inequality came up in every interview as a foundational cause of health disparities in Black and Indigenous communities and other communities of color. Policy was—and remains—the main driver in codifying economic inequity, as it establishes the structures for the ways in which the United States operates and determines "who" has access to "what" and "when." Structural racism has been a factor on the front-end of developing policies that shape economic structures and access to wealth, wielded as a weapon against non-White communities via restrictive covenants, redlining, zoning, disinvestment, tribal nation termination and more, resulting in the cumulative growth over generations of racial wealth gaps. Breaking down these longstanding structural inequities and building equitable economic policy, interviewees said, is vital.

Reparations came up in several interviews as another essential action to build economic justice. The interviewee who provided the previous quote is not Black and came to their understanding of the necessity of reparations from their stronger grasp of the level of devastation from lost—and stolen— wealth creation of Black communities. They described how wealth creation must be addressed head-on, not only as a means of economic repair, but also as a significant lever to positively impact health outcomes.

They also shared an example of how reparations are a part of a larger strategy that addresses one of the social determinants of health: the nascent Evanston Reparations Project in Illinois is the first of its kind in the country to attempt reparations for Black Americans.

A final, recurring theme amongst interviewees was the need for a living wage, universal basic income, and other forms of opportunity for those whom the current economic system marginalizes.

Economic justice appeared in the literature scan, too, including the need to transition local and regional economies to rise to the demands of a climate-resilient and equitable future (Governor of California, Office of Planning and Research 2021). The literature also pointed out that economic justice looks for ways to diverge from the common practice of profits over people: "Addressing the root cause of an extractive economy creates a local model for community governance, centers communities of color most impacted by environmental racism as decision-makers of their energy resources, and respects the Earth and our ecosystem" (Obias and Yoko-Young 2020).

3. Power and Decision-Making Authority

Movement building and collective action are among the most vital levers for local change. We heard repeatedly from interviewees the strong desire to expand the scope of investment in all aspects of collective action and mobilization so communities can achieve real, sustained change. In short, invest money, time, and people resources in movement building.

Throughout the literature scan, we found that community work was accomplished in coalition and partnership, rather than independently and disjointedly. Movement building is a key lever to sustainable local change, by and for the people who are oppressed by structural racism. Communities used movement-building levers most often while working to build trust and implement place-based solutions.

According to the Ford Foundation, only 5 percent of racial equity funding in the US is specifically focused on movement building and grassroots organizing. In contrast, our interviews and literature review regularly highlighted the vital need for movement building and collective action in achieving community-led policy change. Ultimately, interviewees repeatedly said, communities don't need expert opinions; they need philanthropy's collective trust in their chosen solutions.

The literature showed that movement building, policy, and funding are often part of a trifecta. Interviewees advised investment in coalition building at all levels within philanthropy.

Funding processes maintain unequal systems of power and need to be democratized. Interviewees and literature called for the democratization of the grantmaking process, meaning that funders and grantees (including intermediaries' grantees) would be engaged in conversation to reexamine and redefine where, who, and how to fund. Other stated examples of power sharing include co-creating the design, implementation, and evaluation of grantmaking (e.g., participatory grantmaking); reexamining and redefining reporting processes and impact assessments; and participatory convenings and conferences in which agendas are co-created with community grantees within a framework of shared values.

In other work that Metropolitan Group is doing with philanthropic grantees, we hear an overwhelming call for trust-based philanthropy, including multi-year unrestricted funding, streamlined applications and reporting, and a commitment to building relationships based on transparency, dialogue, and mutual learning. One interviewee recommended

Pisces Foundation Mosaic Momentum Initiative as an example of this power-sharing model of grantmaking.

In short, community leaders and organizations want authentic collaboration and an overall democratization of the grantmaking model to be not only responsive to but also designed with—if not guided by—communities. Community engagement requires a willingness to rethink the ways philanthropies structure their staffing models, amongst other structural amendments, but it is very possible and strongly desired.

Shared values—defined by community—must motivate and drive local action. The literature reinforces the evidence for community-driven solutions (and the flexible grantmaking parameters that must accompany community-defined work). Local program funding must ensure that impacted communities define outcomes (including what it means to thrive) and drive the design and implementation of solutions for themselves, with space to work in creative and effective ways.

When a solution is anchored in the community's values, and the community has helped design the solution—versus enacting a solution dictated by a funder or intermediary—the change is more likely to take hold.

Multiple problems require multisolving. According to climate expert Elizabeth Sawin, multisolving is when people pool expertise, funding, and political will to solve multiple problems with a single investment of time and money. It's an approach with great relevance in this era of complex, interlinked, social, and environmental challenges. In fact, the most common theme in the literature review was the need for multiple approaches to addressing climate justice and equity.

Simply put, because climate change is a threat multiplier, it demands creative and flexible solutions, from green infrastructure (UCSF Fielding School of Public Health 2020) to economic justice (Community Wealth 2021) to clean energy (City of Portland 2018) to accessible water (White-Newsome 2020). As reflected in the literature review, community planning, trust-building, and place-based activities are the most common combination of multisolving solutions that communities are using to address climate justice and equity.

Addressing the structural or social determinants of health, such as employment or earning a livable wage, might not look at face value like a climate solution or a racial justice solution. Yet these areas need support to break down the economic barriers that limit access to health.

Better local data—and support to effectively use it—is a priority to spur needed change. Interviewees identified Community-Based Participatory Research (CBPR) as an essential component to truly understand structural inequalities, as well as the solutions that have the highest probability of eliminating them, specific to each place. This form of research includes validation from the ground, which positions the research as recognizable, trusted, and more likely to be used. As one interviewee put it, "Those closest to the pain are clearest about the solutions."

We also heard the need for capacity building to use new technologies to support local and regional data collection, assessment, and use to make the case for local policy change, including effective data visualization to show where change needs to happen first. This was particularly notable in the climate-related literature review, where environmental monitoring tools, such as EJSCREEN, My Environment, and other technology solutions, are being or can be used to quantify climate impacts on the health of communities.

Many interviewees pointed out that a shift is needed in conceptions of what data to trust—and specifically who is an expert, what is evidence, and who and what is "legitimate." "Nonprofits and foundations prioritize research and data," says one interviewee. "But people with lived experience are often not recognized as having legitimate knowledge. We look at how we can lift them up in our work."

Youth voices, power, and leadership are already prevalent forces in climate conversations; additional investment to amplify and build their leadership is highly desired. Youth voices on climate change are vital, say many of our interviewees, noting that young people have grown up in an era where they expect racial justice, have a vision for a healthier country and world, and have to live with the long-term impact of a changing climate. But the cadre of youth who are most supported, promoted, and visible don't adequately represent the nation. "Who is speaking for young people?" asks one interviewee. "It can't just be Greta [Thunberg]. We need young voices of color."

Several items in our literature review pointed out that education systems and curricula are powerful levers for change, and there is a need for curricula that connect climate, racial justice, and health to disrupt current assumptions and narratives. From an article in K12 by student Ndidi Opara: "[T]o meaningfully discuss climate change, we need to understand that climate change affects some more than others and must be addressed with intersectionality. This understanding of climate justice for all is what has been missing in our conversations."

4. Narrative

Narratives are the aggregation of stories and experiences that shape shared ideas about the world and why things are the way they are. Both literature and interviewees note that narrative change is a driving factor in mindset, culture shift, and policy change. Structural racism, says the narrative initiative, has kept the white supremacy narrative intact. For this reason, we treat the narrative landscape as a structure.

Constructive narratives are anchored in values of inclusion and strength. As we mapped narratives that emerged across the social media scan, literature review, and interviews, the dominant themes included inclusion, interdependence, and collective benefit (Figure 9.1).

For example, Anat Shenker-Osorio, one of the creators of the Race Class Narrative Project, advised in a *New York Times* story on talking about race to

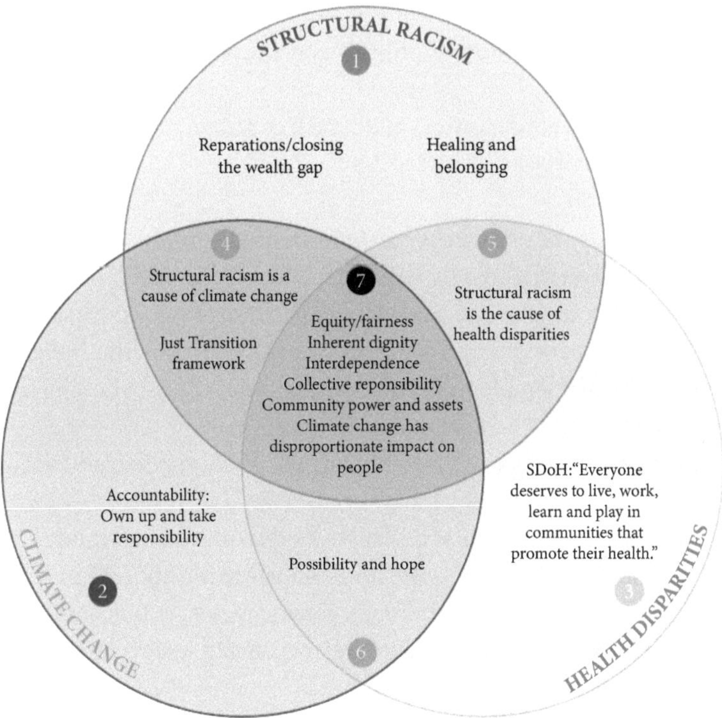

Figure 9.1 Constructive or helpful narrative themes

"begin by naming a shared value with deliberate reference to race, describe the problem as one of deliberate division or racial scapegoating, and then close with how the policy . . . will mean better well-being or justice or freedom for all working people" (Edsall 2021).

An interdependence narrative, said one interviewee, may also be the best approach to fear-based counter-narratives: "People are so lost, with no collective outlet; the message of fear brings them together. Messages of hope, solidarity and collectivism are out there, but they're not good about punching through every day."

Interviewees and the literature suggested other important values to explore, including:

- thriving;
- healing and belonging;
- curiosity;
- hope and possibility;
- the inherent worthiness of all people;
- history, including the history and assets of communities that create strength and the history of policies and decisions that create oppression; and
- alignment with conservative values, such as security, authority, sanctity, prosperity, liberty, and stewardship.

Damaging narratives are anchored in individualism and protect structural racism. Overwhelmingly, the literature—and many interviews—focused on how existing narratives (including within public health) continue to fault individual behavior and suggest that people of color and Indigenous people are more vulnerable to health risks, without directly linking this to conditions caused by structural racism (Figure 9.2).

The narrative around COVID-19 has provided a mini case study, as Color of Change discusses in Building Narrative Power: "COVID . . . was a great opportunity to illuminate structural causes for disparate impact, and in many cases the narrative did that. But much of the narrative still reinforced personal blame . . . Instead, (we should) perpetuate messages that shine a light upon policies and historical legacies that negatively impact the health of Black communities" (Robinson 2018).

Indeed, the Collaborative on Media and Messaging reports that public understanding of structural racism as a driver of health inequity has not

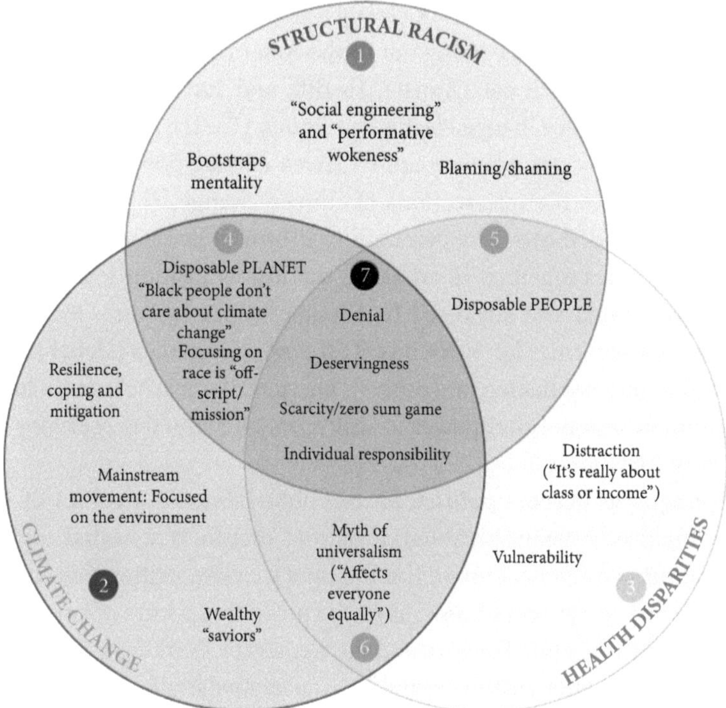

Figure 9.2 Damaging or harmful narrative themes

increased during COVID-19, and calls on communicators to "make those connections, tell stories that illustrate them, give concrete examples of their implications, and suggest solutions to address the structural factors that contribute to health inequity."

A consistent, shared narrative linking climate, structural racism, and health is not dominant. One interviewee articulated the complexity and inconsistency in efforts to intertwine the three issues. "Climate justice folks say we must lift racism," they said. "The broader climate movement wants to frame the issues as 'climate change impacts everyone' because they don't want to turn people off." They even noted that in a recent issue of *The Lancet*, the equity focus got buried because some partners wanted to lead with "impacts everyone," then add "some more than others."

Shenker-Osorio, again in the *New York Times*, points out that this "dependent clause" messaging doesn't work. "For many people of color, this feels like race is an afterthought. For many whites, it feels like a non sequitur," she said (Edsall 2021).

Some of the most focused work clearly linking climate, structural racism and health appears to be coming out of the American Public Health Association (APHA) Center for Climate, Health, and Equity, and the Kresge Foundation's Climate Change Health and Equity (CCHE) program. CCHE seeks to help advocates advance equity-driven climate policies, using messaging that frames the intersections of climate change, racial justice, and health equity and shows why community-driven policies are needed that tackle these issues together. In addition, the Just Transition Framework—collectively created and advanced by Climate Justice Alliance, Movement Strategy Center, Center for Story Based Strategy, Grassroots Global Justice, the EDGE Funders Alliance, and others—also intertwines the three in its call for "economic and political power to shift from an extractive economy to a regenerative economy."

Language has become politicized and polarizing. As a subset of narratives, nuance of language about structural racism is a heated topic of conversation and scholarship. In just the time we were writing this chapter, numerous articles[1] appeared describing the polarizing nature of language. A fall 2021 poll by Jacobin, YouGov, and the Center for Working-Class Politics found that "race is undeniably vexing." This narrative itself—that there is no simple answer in a deeply divided country—leaves many who want to discuss structural racism afraid to speak up or pessimistic that the debate will move beyond hollow or performative words.

For those working in conservative contexts, several studies indicate that using overt language, like *structural racism*, may create a wedge in the conversation. Frameworks Institute advised using language like *fairness* and *people getting what they need* and describing rather than naming the effects of structural racism, for example, showing how policies can ensure (or prevent) resources flowing more fairly into neighborhoods and zip codes (Sweetland 2021). Metropolitan Group's work in 2016 with Voices for Healthy Kids landed on a targeted universalism approach (aim to help everyone, starting where the need is greatest and then expanding); a 2020 update to that work that is more overt about structural racism is proving challenging for advocates in conservative states to use. One interviewee added that the term *structural* can mean "big government policy" to some more conservative thinkers, who may prefer entrepreneurial approaches and value dignity and freedom.

---

[1] The Absurd Side of the Social Justice Industry; The AMA Embraces Leftist Language; Paging Dr. Orwell. The American Medical Association Takes on the Politics of Language.

Is it more important, one interviewee asked, "to ensure racially equitable outcomes by doing the work in a particular way that ensures that people of color receive the outcomes? Or to continue talking about and naming racism explicitly and showing how we got here?"

Narrative authority must rest in communities. Evidence points to the vital role of community-driven narratives. One interviewee used the term *narrative authority*, meaning the power of communities experiencing the impact of structural racism to define, drive, and own their own narratives. That theme repeated across the research: "There should be investments in people telling their own stories as well as the PhDs with higher levels of formal education who can provide another level of analysis," said one interviewee.

Evidence for effective actions to respect and strengthen narrative authority include:

- ***Community storytelling.*** Specific stories from people and communities experiencing structural racism—illuminating both historical context and current reality—must be told across many mediums and channels. Rather than create messages for communities to use, foundations can fund organizations—led by and working with those closest to the problem and closest to the strengths—to gather, tell, and amplify stories. One interviewee offered the example of the Soros Justice Fellowship supporting Michelle Alexander to write *The New Jim Crow.*

  Clear stories that directly connect climate impact, structural racism, and health outcomes—from communities' perspective—can shift dominant narratives and serve other objectives, including illuminating inequitable structures and health impacts; demonstrating the deep connection between Indigenous communities, the health of the land and the health of the people; amplifying leadership and solutions from within communities; and demonstrating interconnection.

- ***Community power and mobilizing.*** Not only do community-driven stories shift the narrative *about* communities, the act of storytelling also builds power by increasing self-efficacy and mobilizing action. Several interviewees stated that communities most impacted often don't know the full history of why things are the way they are; this is especially true regarding climate change. In the words of one interviewee, "There is a certain power that comes with knowing that something is not wrong with you. We're interested in narrative strategy in the sense that communities of color can use these stories to become empowered about what they're fighting for."

Other interviewees echoed this idea that narrative change is often best paired with organizing efforts—and in fact must be. "The level of contempt and devaluation coming from Congress of everyone who does not look like them is incredibly high, and no narrative is going to shift it," said one interviewee. "That narrative work needs to be accompanied by political will, which is only achieved through robust civic engagement."

- ***Community-designed narrative strategies and infrastructure.*** Color of Change defines narrative infrastructure as "the set of systems we maintain in order to exercise narrative power, which is the ability to change the norms and rules our society lives by reliably over time." The California Endowment emphasizes that rather than building a new infrastructure to support narrative change, or build up their own infrastructure, funders should instead "help to embed narrative change capacity in existing social movements and coalitions."

  For example, one interviewee cited The Center for Story-Based Strategy, which ensures frontline communities have the resources they need to advance their own narratives. Foundations can also strengthen organizations' narrative capacity and infrastructure, including staffing and rapid response resources (Lynn and Kathlene 2020).

For foundations working on racial equity programs, narrative is elemental. "We can't just say, 'do this.' People have to make sense of it," said one interviewee.

Some specific actions mentioned in the literature and interviews include boldly naming and describing the impact of structural racism on health in social media, media statements, and other communications; amplifying clear and specific stories of conditions and change needed; amplifying stories of people changing systems, including their paths to a solution; and supporting journalists to tell more accurate stories, including the *why* behind the story from a structural racism perspective.

Narrative understanding, infrastructure and capacity is needed in philanthropy, public health, and healthcare. Healing Through Policy, an initiative of the de Beaumont Foundation, APHA, and the National Collaborative for Health Equity, recommends several strategies for narrative action, including issuing executive orders, resolutions, ordinances, and declarations to advance racial equity (deBeaumont 2021). This has been a trend over the past few years as organizations, cities, and states declare racism as a public health crisis; the level of action and impact varies. Other organizations, including Voices for Healthy Kids and the American Psychological Association are taking these declarations one step further by naming their own role in upholding structural racism and being accountable for change. As statements of both kinds continue to emerge, one interviewee suggested that this may be a space for capacity building to ensure that organizations fulfill their stated commitments and are equipped to withstand dog-whistle criticism.

There is also a need to continue building capacity within the public health and philanthropy fields to stop using harmful data, messages, and narratives, and instead to increasingly name, illustrate, and address structural racism. Open Societies Foundation calls the current narrative surrounding the public health system "steeped in racism" for blaming individuals for making "poor lifestyle choices" and suggesting that oppressed and marginalized communities are responsible for their own health problems.

Health Affairs boldly exposed this blind spot in a series of editorials in 2020. "Despite racism's alarming impact on health and the wealth of scholarship that outlines its ill effects, preeminent scholars and the journals that publish them, including *Health Affairs*, routinely fail to interrogate racism as a critical driver of racial health inequities," the editorial team wrote, offering new standards for publishing on racial health inequities.

Finding 3: Climate Change Is an Existential Threat to Human Health, Exacerbated by Structural Racism

Climate change is the biggest threat to health, as described by the World Health Organization, and is exacerbated by structural racism in three ways:

- It creates inequitable conditions in communities of color and Indigenous communities—in housing, economic stability, health, and many other factors. It creates "sacrifice zones" where the ravages of floods, poor air quality, vector-borne diseases, wildfires, extreme heat, drought, and other deadly effects of climate change hit harder and more frequently—and where residents lack the economic resources to escape, relocate and thrive through disasters. The same families that experience one climate disaster after another are the families disproportionately faced with structural barriers to access health, wellbeing, and equity.

- It upholds environmental racism, which includes racial discrimination in environmental policymaking, in the enforcement of regulations and laws, in the deliberate targeting of communities of color for toxic waste disposal and the siting of polluting industries, and in the history of excluding people of color and Indigenous people from mainstream environmental groups, decision-making boards, commissions, and regulatory bodies.
- It exacerbates climate change itself by upholding structures, systems, and mindsets that are grounded in white supremacy, that devalue communities of color and Indigenous communities, and that maintain a transactional relationship with nature as a resource to be harnessed and depleted.

Structural racism creates many factors that influence an individual's or community's ability to adapt to climate change. At the individual (or biological) level, age, illness, and disease can jeopardize a person's ability to escape or adapt to climate change and to stay healthy or recover from illness. Social factors, the social determinants of health like affordable transportation, quality housing, and linguistic and social cohesion, create conditions that grant or deny communities opportunities to survive or thrive in the aftermath of a climate event.

These factors are influenced by root causes, such as racial segregation, generational poverty and economic disinvestment, community violence, and discrimination, which create additional barriers. One report clearly stated that "structural and institutional racism in our economic, government and social systems has resulted and continues to result in the disproportionate distribution of the benefits and burdens of our society leading to increased climate risk" (Yuen et al. 2017).

Finding 4: The Way Funders Act Is as Powerful as How They Fund

Funders centering health equity must "walk the walk" in internal systems, processes, practices, and culture and the makeup and behaviors of their board, staff, and leadership. Transformative action needs to include a consistent, transparent, integrated process for interrogating, refining, and, in some cases, dismantling institutional barriers. The work of eliminating structural racism and positively impacting health and well-being demands at all levels a staff that is educated, enlightened, and aligned. It also demands a common language and definitions of key terminology—including a definition of structural racism.

Other considerations include the makeup of researchers and evaluators and definitions of expertise and evidence; (ease or burden of) grantmaking processes and practices; the organization's internal culture and the experience grantees and others have interacting with it; and the way funders signal either a supporting role (e.g., studying and funding from afar) or an identity as a committed ally (e.g., volunteering for racial justice, social justice, and health equity organizations; serving on their boards; listening and learning in community-led spaces).

The conception of evidence, expert, and leadership must be radically reimagined and broadened. Many interviewees expressed the desire for an expanded definition of evidence and "expert opinion." Specifically, the lived experience of those whom the system most negatively impacts must be a valued part of developing strategies to address issues impacting said communities.

Interviewees called for a commitment to recognize community leaders—specifically people who are directly engaged in the work *in addition* to those grasstops leaders and experts who are nationally recognized and can speak to the work. Both are needed, yet funders too often overlook those closest to the ground. Moreover, funders must compensate community experts participating in focus groups, convenings, speaking engagements, and other encounters at the same level they compensate academic experts. Too often, these invitations (or requests) are extended without adequate compensation, but because of the power imbalance between organization and funder, community-based organization leaders feel uncomfortable saying no.

Interviewees further suggested funders require academic institutions they fund to compensate those community members with whom they engage or partner. This, they say, will go far in laying the groundwork for authentic trust building by helping to shift the power paradigm that currently exists.

> "You're a university … huge difference in infrastructure and power … value the community and their cultural knowledge systems."
>
> —Interviewee

Relationships of trust must be built on deep engagement and shared power.
Among interviewees, there was tremendous energy for funders to build
relationships and meaningfully engage with communities.

> "[A]ny significant change has to be a bottom-up solution. Top down has
> failed."
>
> —Interviewee

This was strongly reiterated in the literature, which called for "building up
movements before you stand up tables" (Chlala and Said 2021). There is evidence for the value of common or shared spaces, supported but not managed
by funders, where community dialogue can spark local learning, healing, and
actions based on community identified needs; can build shared capacity;
and can result in aligned goals based on deeply shared values.

Several interviewees echoed the need for an intentional space for funders to be positioned in a *listening*, learning, and receiving stance. "Start
with listening, not just so you can capture information, but listen so you
can play it back to the persons who are talking because they don't have a
history of being listened to," said one interviewee. "Working folks rarely get
an opportunity to be in a public space where people are interested in their
imagination, interested in their vision, interested in their thoughts about the
future."

Physical presence and active, authentic engagement with communities is
essential for trust to develop. Being shoulder-to-shoulder with those most
impacted creates real opportunities for philanthropic staff and leadership
to listen, embody solidarity, and learn to yield power. Without deep listening and interest in local voices, funding distribution can replay existing
power dynamics. Nearly every one of our 19 interviewees elevated this
point, and we read it across the literature scan. Clearly stated, the paradigm
that "the funder is always right because they have the money" is being
challenged. The relationship between philanthropy and grantees is interdependent, and thus requires true, transparent, and authentic collaboration
and partnership to be impactful in the stated goal of eliminating structural
barriers.

Once relationships, and trust, have been fostered, deeper engagement can
begin. An example of an existing, successful approach highlighted in an

interview is RWJF's engagement with the Neighborhood Funders Group (NFG) and its Amplify Fund. This is an approach to place-based engagement that centers the voices of Black, Indigenous and communities of color.

> "[P]eople who have been victims of racism must be in positions of equitable decision-making. That's the only way to break the cycle."
>
> —Interviewee

One example of rich community-led engagement came from the New Mexico Energy Transition Action. This policy was initially introduced without the community's engagement and input and had a problematic framework and language. Community leadership stepped up to form a community coalition, which launched a health impact assessment in partnership with the University of New Mexico Tree Center. The health impact assessment—an example of participatory action research—was designed to directly consult the community being assessed, and included key health indicators initially omitted, such as cultural and spiritual health, as well as connection to the land. Ultimately, the New Mexico Energy Transition Act was passed with the support and buy-in of the community.

Recommendations

Drawing from the key findings and comprehensive input, and layering in expertise from Metropolitan Group's team, we offer the following recommendations to inform the shift to centering racial equity:

1. To meaningfully address structural racism, funders must change internal structures.
2. To meaningfully address structural racism funders must change external structures by using their voice on each of the four structures described in our findings and by funding organizations and movements working on structural changes.
3. Funders who want to impact health should commit to investing in climate justice—centered in relationships and community power.

Next Steps: Bold Action

There is anticipation and hope among the people we interviewed for the shift to centering racial equity. There is evidence from communities about what is needed to address structural racism and health and climate change and health. There is clearly a role for philanthropy to play in how it acts, how and what it funds, and how it uses its power and voice.

To paraphrase many of our interviewees: "Stop talking about it and *be about it.*"

Acknowledgements

Thank you to Erica Ellis, Eric Friedenwald-Fishman, Max Friedenwald-Fishman, Shadiin Garcia, Kirsten Gunst, Kelly Hilovsky, Aayaan Jamwal, Kevin Kirkpatrick, Thomas Price Lang, and Vernice Miller-Travis for your valuable contributions to this chapter.

Bibliography

1% for the Planet. 2020. *Nonprofits fighting for social and environmental justice.* June 19, 2020. https://www.onepercentfortheplanet.org/stories/nonprofits-fighting-for-social-environmental-justice.

Alcalde G. How to develop a strong vision to deepen a nonprofit's impact. *Mainebiz.* October 4, 2021. https://www.mainebiz.biz/article/how-to-develop-a-strong-vision-to-deepen-a-nonprofits-impact.

American Medical Association and Center for Health Justice. 2021. *Advancing health equity: A guide to language, narrative and concepts.* https://www.ama-assn.org/system/files/ama-aamc-equity-guide.pdf.

Ayala R. Community-led clean energy strategies. *The American Council for an Energy-Efficient Economy.* October 21, 2021. https://storymaps.arcgis.com/stories/88cd8a715089418890d9ec4d09a25648.

California Environmental Justice Alliance. Defining environmental justice communities: Using CalEnviroScreen in state policy. *Medium,* September 6, 2019. https://cejapower.medium.com/defining-environmental-justice-communities-using-calenviroscreen-in-state-policy-4d1f350b3207.

California Public Utilities Commission. *Environmental and social justice plan version 2.0 draft for public input.* October 26, 2021. https://www.cpuc.ca.gov/-/media/cpuc-website/divisions/news-and-outreach/documents/news-office/key-issues/esj/draft-cpuc-esj-2010262021c.pdf.

Cha MJ, Pastor M. *A roadmap to a low carbon future: Four pillars for a just transition. Climate Equity Network.* April 2019. https://dornsife.usc.edu/assets/sites/242/docs/Just_Transition_Final_Report_2019.pdf.

Chlala R, Said N, eds. Building power in place—Nashville: Reshaping the city towards an economy for all. *Neighborhood Funders Group*. February 25, 2021. https://nfg.org/building-power-in-place-nashville-reshaping-the-city-towards-an-economy-for-all/.

City of Portland. About PCEF. *Portland Clean Energy Community Benefits Fund*. Accessed 2018. https://www.portland.gov/bps/cleanenergy/about.

Community Wealth. *The Cleveland model: How the evergreen cooperatives are building community wealth*. 2021. https://community-wealth.org/content/cleveland-model-how-evergreen-cooperatives-are-building-community-wealth.

De Beaumont Foundation. Healing through policy: Creating pathways to racial justice. *Policy and Practice Briefs*. 2021. https://debeaumont.org/programs/healing-through-policy/.

Detroiters Working for Environmental Justice. "From the bottom up: Climate action in Detroit." Video. January 25, 2021. https://www.youtube.com/watch?v=tfiy4djZoNM%t=5s.

Dobens C. New York City Council passes legislation to help protect our children, communities, and climate by transitioning to electric school buses. *WE ACT*. October 7, 2021. https://www.weact.org/2021/10/new-york-city-council-passes-legislation-to-protect-our-children-communities-climate-by-transitioning-to-electric-school-buses/.

Donors of Color: Climate Funder's Justice Pledge. To Solve the Climate Crisis, We Need Funders to Change the Way They Do Business. 2021. https://climate.donorsofcolor.org/.

Emerald Cities Collaborative and People Organizing to Demand Environmental & Economic Rights (PODER). *Climate equity and community engagement in building electrification: A toolkit*. November 10, 2020. https://emeraldcities.org/wp-content/uploads/2021/05/Climate-Equity-and-Community-Engagement-Toolkit_Nov102020.pdf.

Environmental Protection Agency. 2021. Justice40 climate and economic justice screening tool and Executive Order 12898 revisions. *White House Environmental Justice Advisory Council*. May 13, 2021. https://www.epa.gov/sites/default/files/2021-05/documents/whejac_interim_final_recommendations_0.pdf.

Fallon C. New York City students confront climate change impacts and explore resilient solutions. *The National Wildlife Federation*. October 11, 2021. https://nwf.org/Home/Latest-News/Press-Releases/2021/10-11-21-RiSC-Coney-Island.

Gómez CA, Kleinman DV, Pronk N, Gordon GLW, Ochiai E, Blakey C, Johnson A, Brewer KH. Addressing health equity and social determinants of health through healthy people 2030. *Journal of Public Health Management and Practice*. 2021;27(6):249–257. doi: 10.1097/PHH.0000000000001297

Governor of California, Office of Planning and Research. *Governor Newsom proposes $750 million to build economic resilience in the face of climate change*. May 14, 2021. https://opr.ca.gov/news/2021/05-14.html.

Governor of New York. Governor Hochul announces new statewide community air monitoring initiative, first of its kind in the U.S. September 21, 2021. https://www.governor.ny.gov/news/governor-hochul-announces-new-statewide-community-air-monitoring-initiative-first-its-kind-us.

Greenlink Analytics. *Visualizing data through neighborhood equity maps*. 2020. https://www.greenlinkanalytics.org/gem.

Gupta, Shalini. Climate change, health, and equity survey findings: Gaps, needs, and opportunities. *Health and Environmental Funders Network*. March 2020. https://hefn.org/giving-insight/2020-hefn-year-in-review/.

HBCU Green Fund. Environmental justice leader Mustafa Ali to dialogue with White House advisor Gina McCarthy at BIPOC climate justice virtual event. *Send2Press*. April 8, 2021. https://www.send2press.com/wire/environmental-justice-leader-mustafa-ali-to-dialogue-with-white-house-advisor-gina-mccarthy-at-bipoc-climate-justice-virtual-event/.

Junod A, Martin C, Marx R, Rogin A. *Equitable investments in resilience: A review of benefit-cost analysis in federal flood mitigation infrastructure.* Urban Institute, June 2021. https://www.urban.org/sites/default/files/publication/104302/equitable-investments-in-resilience.pdf

Kelly C, Reta M. Implementing Biden's Justice40 commitment to combat environmental racism. Center for *American Progress*, June 22, 2021. https://www.americanprogress.org/article/implementing-bidens-justice40-commitment-combat-environmental-racism/.

King County Climate Action Team. *Making King County more resilient, sustainable and equitable: 2020 strategic climate action plan.* Accessed December 3, 2021. https://kingcounty.gov/services/environment/climate/actions-strategies/strategic-climate-action-plan.aspx.

KLRN, SciTechNow. *Community solutions to climate change.* Video, PBS. March 2, 2018. https://www.pbs.org/video/community-solutions-climate-change-4qdcbz/.

Little Village Environmental Justice Organization. *Coal power plant shutdown.* Accessed December 2, 2021. http://www.lvejo.org/our-accomplishments/coal-plant-shutdown/.

Lynn J, Kathlene L. "Narrative Change for Health & Racial Equity: Exploring Capacity & Alignment." Prepared on behalf of the California Endowment. October 2020.

Martin C, McTarnaghan S. Institutionalizing urban resilience. *Urban Institute*, December 6, 2018. https://www.urban.org/research/publication/institutionalizing-urban-resilience.

Montgomery M, Blanchard P. Testing justice: New ways to address environmental inequalities. *The Solutions Journal.* 2021. https://thesolutionsjournal.com/testing-justice-new-ways-to-address-environmental-inequalities/.

Edsall T. *The New York Times.* "Should Biden Empadded thhasize Race or Class or Both or None of the Above?" April 28, 2021. https://www.nytimes.com/2021/04/28/opinion/biden-democrats-race-class.html.

Obias L, Yoko-Young E. Energy democracy: Honoring the past and investing in a new energy economy. *Race Forward*, May 5, 2021. https://www.raceforward.org/research/reports/energy-democracy-honoring-past-and-investing-new-energy-economy.

Ohio Environmental Council. *Cleveland comprehensive environmental policy platform: A Vision for 2021–2025.* December 17, 2020. https://theoec.org/news-and-information/clevelandenviropolicyplatform/.

Otosi K. Promoting equitable climate adaptation through community engagement. *Community Development Innovation Review.* Federal Reserve Bank of San Francisco. October 17, 2019. https://www.frbsf.org/community-development/publications/community-development-investment-review/2019/october/promoting-equitable-climate-adaptation-through-community-engagement/.

Partnership for Southern Equity. *Health equity assessment guide.* 2021. https://psequity.org/wp-content/uploads/2021/09/PSE-Earth-Fund-Grant-Release-9_6_21_final.pdf.

Partnership for Southern Equity. *Partnership for Southern Equity receives Bezos Earth Fund grant: Funding will support initiative to curb the global climate crisis.* September 8, 2021. https://psequity.org/wp-content/uploads/2021/09/PSE-Earth-Fund-Grant-Release-9_6_21_final.pdf.

Puget Sound Sage. Powering the transition: Community priorities for a renewable and equitable future. June 2020. https://pugetsoundsage.org/research/climate-justice/community-energy/.

Robinson R. Changing Our Narrative about Narrative: The Infrastructure Require for Building Narrative Power. Color of Change. 2018. https://www.rashadrobinson.com/narrativepower

Root T. He's the youngest Chief in his First Nation's history. Now he's leading their fight against climate change. *Washington Post.* November 8, 2021. https://www.washingtonpost.com/climate-solutions/interactive/2021/climate-change-chief-dana-tizya-tramm/.

Seattle City Council. *Resolution 31757, Version 1.* May 8, 2019. https://clerk.seattle.gov/search/resolutions/31757.

State of New Jersey. *Attorney General Grewal, DEP Acting Commissioner LaTourette announce nine new environmental enforcement actions, seven in environmental justice communities.* 2021.

Sweeney E. "We need to protect communities hit 'first and worst' by climate change, state lawmakers say." *Business Insider.* September 21, 2021. https://www.businessinsider.com/environmental-justice-solutions-protect-low-income-communities-of-color-2021-9.

Sweetland J. Reframing childhood adversity: Promoting upstream approaches. *Frameworks Institute.* 2021. https://www.frameworksinstitute.org/resources/reframing-childhood-adversity-promoting-upstream-approaches/.

Surdna Foundation. *Surdna joins the climate funders pledge.* February 5, 2021. https://surdna.org/news-insights/surdna-joins-the-climate-funders-justice-pledge/.

Tilghman L. How donors can help advance climate justice. *Giving Compass.* July 18, 2021. https://www.givingcompass.org/article/how-donors-can-help-advance-climate-justice/.

Torres, Gerald. Finally, a chance for environmental justice. *Earth Day.* January 15, 2021. https://www.earthday.org/finally-a-chance-for-environmental-justice/.

UCSF Fielding School of Public Health Center for Healthy Climate Solutions. *Parks and green spaces improve community health and reduce health inequities.* November 20, 2020. https://healthyclimatesolutions.org/2020/11/20/parks-and-green-spaces-improve-community-health-and-reduce-health-inequalities/.

United Nations Environment Programme. Plastic pollution is an environmental injustice to vulnerable communities—new report. March 30, 2021. https://www.unep.org/news-and-stories/press-release/plastic-pollution-environmental-injustice-vulnerable-communities-new.

United States Environmental Protection Agency. Resources for creating healthy, sustainable, and equitable communities. Accessed November 30, 2021. https://19january2021snapshot.epa.gov/environmentaljustice/resources-creating-healthy-sustainable-and-equitable-communities_.html.

Vaghul K. Carbon inequities, climate change and complementary solutions. Washington Center for Equitable Growth. February 25, 2016. https://equitablegrowth.org/carbon-inequities-climate-change-and-complementary-solutions/

Vogel J, Carney KM, Smith JB, Herrick C, Stults M, O'Grady M, St. Juliana A, Hosterman H, Giangola L. Climate adaptation: The state of practice in U.S. communities. *Kresge Foundation.* November 1, 2016. https://kresge.org/wp-content/uploads/2020/06/climate-adaptation-the-state-of-practice-in-us-communities-full-report.pdf.

White-Newsome JL. Initiative takes on water systems, climate change, and inequity. *Water Online.* July 15, 2020. https://www.wateronline.com/doc/initiative-takes-on-water-systems-climate-change-and-inequity-0001.

White-Newsome JL. A climate equity agenda informed by community brilliance. *Issues in Science and Technology.* 2021;38(1). https://issues.org/climate-change-equity-community-partnership-white-newsome.

Yuen T, Yurkovich E, Grabowski L, Altshuler B. Guide to equitable community-driven climate preparedness planning. *Urban Sustainability Directors Network.* May 2017. https://www.usdn.org/uploads/cms/documents/usdn_guide_to_equitable_community-driven_climate_preparedness-_high_res.pdf.

Conclusion

As the nine papers in this volume make clear, achieving health equity is impossible until structural racism is recognized as a persistent force that creates inequity and must be addressed and solved. That message propels RWJF to act boldly, moving beyond data and documentation, to pursue evidence-based action. Inequity has been a defining characteristic of the United States since before its formal founding and the need for change is more urgent than ever.

At the same time, we understand that a long view is essential, and our strategic change horizon stretches 25 years into the future. It will take a generation to achieve the goals we have set for ourselves: norming research and academic work to build broader and inclusive practices and methods, creating healthy and equitable community conditions, ensuring economic inclusion that promotes family well-being, and putting equitable and accountable public health and healthcare systems in place.

Meeting these goals and achieving our vision of a future where health is no longer a privilege but a right requires strategic thinking to determine which pressure points, on which systems, can generate the most transformative change. RWJF is particularly focused on the levers that influence the cross-cutting systems of government, health science and knowledge, and media and narrative. Importantly, we have also identified key pathways through which researchers, policymakers, funders, and community activists can act against structural racism and its health effects: racial and ethnic disparities in education, employment, and financial strain; healthcare access and quality; housing and neighborhoods; and the judicial system. Together, we have the power to transform the inequitable institutions, systems, and social practices that people intentionally created, and that still exist today.

This framework enables RWJF to focus on root causes. With our partners and colleagues, we are encouraging methodological innovations and new research approaches, broadening our definition of rigorous evidence, honoring lived experiences as a pathway to knowledge, and prioritizing action. We embrace the idea that those most affected by structural racism can be

Claire Gibbons and Alonzo L. Plough, *Conclusion*. In: *Research to Action*. Edited by: Claire Gibbons and Alonzo L. Plough, Oxford University Press. © Robert Wood Johnson Foundation (2026).
DOI: 10.1093/9780197819876.003.0011

leaders in efforts to eliminate it and have committed to the building of community power and promotion of the narrative and mindset changes that make that possible.

RWJF's programmatic initiatives and funding strategies are directed toward the generational goals we have set for ourselves. Deepening our approach to learning is central to what we do. An example is the Partners for Advancing Health Equity Collaborative,[1] led by Thomas LaVeist, Dean of Tulane University Celia Scott Weatherhead School of Public Health and Tropical Medicine. The collaborative seeks cross-sector synergy and aligns efforts in many corners to create the consistency, processes, guidance, and priorities in research necessary to achieve health equity. We are also increasingly committed to community-driven research and solutions, premised on the recognition that those closest to the challenges are best positioned to address them. That commitment is evident in the Indigenous-Led Solutions to Advance Health Equity and Wellbeing,[2] a funding opportunity developed through a partnership of RWJF's Evidence for Action (E4A) program[3] and the Johns Hopkins Center for Indigenous Health[4] to support community-prioritized investigations that will enhance the health and well-being of Indigenous people.

We also need to challenge biases and outdated conventions in academia, which is the impetus behind Health Equity Scholars for Action. This program identifies and supports early-career researchers from historically underrepresented backgrounds who conduct health equity research. Making meaning from the data that these and other scholars collect requires disaggregating information so that critical within-group differences come to light. Members of racial and ethnic communities have diverse socioeconomic backgrounds and life experiences, and effective investments need to reflect that at a granular level. For example, RWJF has recognized that when Asian Americans are inappropriately grouped together as a single community, distinctions necessary to target resources on the populations that most need them are often lost.[5]

---

[1] RWJF. Partners for Advancing Health Equity. https://www.partners4healthequity.org/.

[2] Indigenous-Led Solutions to Advance Health Equity and Wellbeing. https://www.evidenceforaction.org/funding/new-e4a-funding-opportunity-indigenous-led-solutions-advance-health-equity-and-wellbeing.

[3] RWJF Evidence for Action. https://evidenceforaction.org/.

[4] Center for Indigenous Health. https://cih.jhu.edu/.

[5] Kauh TJ, Read JG, Sheitler AJ. The critical role of racial/ethnic data disaggregation for health equity. *Population Research Policy Review* 2021;40(1):1–7. https://pubmed.ncbi.nlm.nih.gov/33437108/.

Another avenue of great interest to RWJF is reparations. Across the country, momentum is building for reparations as a dignity-enhancing way to acknowledge state-facilitated exploitation and redress the resulting resource deprivation. RWJF staff are represented on the New Jersey Reparations Council, which is studying the state's history and connection to the current racial landscape and recommending reparative justice policies.[6] We have also funded the FXB Center for Health and Human Rights at Harvard University to explore the public health case for reparations in service to health equity.[7]

At RWJF, we view these and many other initiatives as part of our strategy to strongly influence leaders across many sectors and disciplines toward a shared goal—unwinding the structural racism that damages health. At the same time, we are trying to "walk the walk," examining our own elite institutional position and pushing for internal changes as we direct our future resources, define our mission, and demonstrate our commitment to equity. In our language, our grantmaking, and our public presence, we have grown bolder because we believe the times demand it. We are so grateful to the contributors to this volume for helping advance our common cause.

---

[6] New Jersey Reparations Council. https://www.njreparationscouncil.org/.
[7] FXB Center for Health and Human Rights, Harvard University. *Can reparations close the racial health gap?* https://fxb.harvard.edu/event/reparationssymposium/.

Acknowledgments

RWJF commissioned this series of papers to inform its future grantmaking strategy. Deliberately reaching beyond our established networks, we sought out contributors from diverse fields, many of whom brought not only innovative thinking to their scholarship but also insights gained from personal experiences with structural racism. We are so grateful for the powerful work of all the researchers whose work we are proud to present in this book.

Turning their nine papers into this volume required the vision and support of many. An Editorial Review Group oversees the development of this series and provides careful commentary and suggestions. Our colleagues in this group are Anita Chandra, RAND Corporation; Sandro Galea, Boston University; Sherry Glied, New York University; and Sarah Humphreville, Oxford University Press.

Special thanks to the team at RWJF who provided essential leadership and support throughout the development of this manuscript: Ketana Bhavsar, Allyn Brooks-LaSure, and, especially, Kristin Silvani.

Finally, thank you for your exceptional contributions, Karyn Feiden and Eman Quotah.

Editors:
Alonzo L. Plough, PhD, MPH
Claire Gibbons, PhD

Index

For the benefit of digital users, indexed terms that span two pages (e.g., 52–53) may, on occasion, appear on only one of those pages.

Tables and figures are indicated by an italic *t* and *f* following the paragraph number.

9 780197 819845